Department of Health and Social Security

Breast Cancer Screening

Report to the Health Ministers
of England, Wales,
Scotland & Northern Ireland
by a working group chaired by
Professor Sir Patrick Forrest

London   Her Majesty's Stationery Office

© Crown copyright 1986
First published 1986
Third impression 1989
ISBN 0 11 321071 X

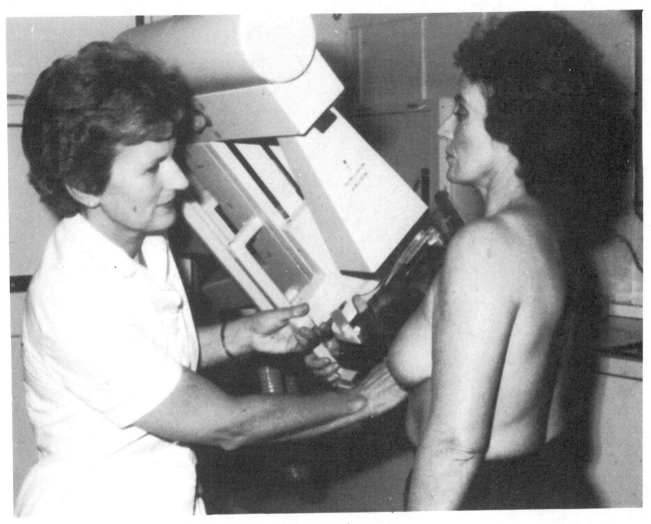

A woman having a mammogram of her breast taken by a radiographer.

Contents

Preface

We were appointed under the Chairmanship of Professor Sir Patrick Forrest in July 1985 by Mr Kenneth Clarke, then Minister for Health, on behalf of all the UK Health Ministers. Our terms of reference were:

i to consider the information now available on breast cancer screening by mammography; the extent to which this suggests necessary changes in UK policy on the provision of mammographic facilities and the screening of symptomless women; and

ii to suggest a range of policy options and assess the benefits and costs associated with them; and set out the service planning, manpower, financial and other implications of implementing such options.

Details of membership are at Annex A.

Our interim report, addressing itself to part one of the remit, was presented to Ministers in January 1986. In this report we concluded that:

'The information that is already available from the principal overseas studies demonstrates that screening by mammography can lead to the prolongation of the lives of women aged 50 and over with breast cancer. There is a convincing case, on clinical grounds, for a change in UK policy on the provision of mammographic facilities and the screening of symptomless women.' And, that,

'The preliminary view of the working group is that it would not be sensible to introduce mammographic screening on a UK basis without providing the necessary back-up services to assess the abnormalities that would be detected'.

After reaching these conclusions we went on to complete the second part of our remit. In all we met on 11 occasions and considered about 70 papers including published papers which are listed in the selected bibliography. Many of our meetings were also attended by co-opted experts who represented other relevant disciplines or were specially invited to present evidence. The names of these experts are at Annex A. In presenting our report we wish to acknowledge with gratitude their invaluable contributions.

We also wish to thank the Scottish Home and Health Department for funding a study to provide specific information on the costs of screening in Edinburgh that we had requested. Finally, we wish to record our gratitude to the Department of Health and Social Security for providing the Secretariat, whose courteous and efficient support greatly facilitated our task.

We present at the end of our report our main conclusions.

November 1986

1   Introduction

Breast cancer

1.1. Breast cancer is the commonest form of cancer among women in the UK. Each year there are approximately 24,000 new cases and 15,000 deaths from the disease. This compares with 75,000 deaths among women from all forms of cancer, and 339,000 deaths among women from all causes (see Annex B, Table B–1). The UK mortality rate is the highest in Western Europe and North America, regions where the disease is generally commoner and mortality rates higher than in the rest of the world (see Annex B, Figure B.1). The disease is rare under the age of 35; between 30 and 34 the incidence and mortality rates in the UK are 19.6 and 5.9 per 100,000 women. By 50–54 these rates have risen to 145.9 and 73.7 per 100,000 women, and they continue to increase with age (see Annex B, Figure B.2).

1.2 Neither the cause of breast cancer nor the means of preventing the disease are known.

1.3 Advances in surgery, radiotherapy, chemotherapy and hormone therapy have achieved only modest increases in survival following treatment. One reason is that the effectiveness of treatment is related to the stage at which the disease presents. In the UK about one third of patients with breast cancer do not present until the tumour is large and often advanced.

1.4 At present, the only way substantially to reduce the number of deaths from the disease is to detect it before the patient presents with symptoms. The value of early detection by mass population screening is best tested by observing whether, in well-conducted controlled trials, fewer women offered screening compared to those not offered screening die at a given age from breast cancer.

Evidence from overseas trials

1.5 The results of two such randomised trials have been reported. In one trial conducted over the past 20 years in New York (a project of the Health Insurance Plan (HIP) of Greater New York) it has been found that, among women aged 40–64 when they were first offered screening, breast cancer mortality was reduced by 30 per cent for up to 10 years. A significant beneficial effect has persisted for at least 18 years. The second more recent trial in the counties of Kopparberg and Ostergötland in Sweden has shown a similar effect over a 9-year follow-up period among women aged 40–74. In both these trials the beneficial effect of screening was concentrated in women aged 50 and over, and an effect on mortality of screening women aged 40–49 is still uncertain.

1.6 Results from two studies in the Netherlands which compared the mortality of screened and unscreened women, showed that the chances of a screened woman dying were between one half and one third of those of an unscreened woman. Thus, even allowing for bias due to the design of these studies, this favourable effect is consistent with the conclusions from the American and Swedish trials that screening could make a substantial impact on breast cancer deaths in women aged 50 and over.

1.7 The evidence from these trials led us to conclude that screening can reduce mortality from breast cancer, although as we discuss in Chapter 5 the reduction varies with the age of the women screened. The effect on overall mortality is necessarily small because the number of deaths from causes other than breast cancer is much greater. The methods used in these trials were X-ray mammography alone or combined with clinical examination. These and other possible methods are described and evaluated in Chapters 3 and 4.

UK Trial of Early Detection of Breast Cancer

1.8 A large, 7-year, multi-centre, population-based trial of regular screening by mammography with clinical examination and by breast self-examination was started in the UK in 1979. In Edinburgh the study was extended by the institution of a randomised controlled trial similar to the HIP and Swedish studies. Although no information on mortality from the UK studies will be available until 1988, detection rates and extent of the disease are similar to those observed at a corresponding stage of the Swedish study. (Descriptions of the overseas and UK trials are given in Annex C).

Mass screening

1.9 Implementing a mass population screening programme is much more complex than organising a trial. No country yet has experience with a successful national breast cancer screening programme on which the UK could draw, although some countries in Western Europe are planning or starting to introduce programmes. In the UK there are already some screening facilities outside the centres participating in the UK Trials, including those provided by voluntary groups, the private medical sector and employers. In addition some health authorities have begun to plan to introduce screening services. Relevant experience has been gained from screening programmes for other diseases, in particular for cervical cancer. We believe that the development of any national programme will require careful planning not only of the basic screening services but also to ensure the availability of the necessary assessment, diagnostic and treatment services for screen-detected abnormalities. Otherwise the full benefit will not be achieved.

2 Principles of screening and their application to breast cancer

2.1 In this report we mean by 'screening' the performance of tests on apparently well women to detect those with unrecognised breast cancer. Principles of screening were first formulated in 1968 by Wilson and Jungner for the World Health Organisation.

In general these principles are:

2.1.1 the condition sought should pose an important health problem;

2.1.2 the natural history of the disease should be well understood;

2.1.3 there should be a recognisable early stage;

2.1.4 treatment of the disease at an early stage should be of more benefit than treatment started at a later stage;

2.1.5 there should be a suitable test;

2.1.6 the test should be acceptable to the population;

2.1.7 there should be adequate facilities for the diagnosis and treatment of abnormalities detected;

2.1.8 for diseases of insidious onset, screening should be repeated at intervals determined by the natural history of the disease;

2.1.9 the chance of physical or psychological harm to those screened should be less than the chance of benefit;

2.1.10 the cost of a screening programme should be balanced against the benefit it provides.

Below we consider the extent to which breast cancer meets these criteria.

Important health problem

2.2 Breast cancer is the commonest cancer affecting British women, and the countries in the United Kingdom have the highest mortality rates from breast cancer in the world. (See Chapter 1 and Annex B). The cause of the disease is not understood and there is no immediate hope of prevention. Survival after treatment is improving but about two thirds of women who develop breast cancer are still likely to die from it.

Natural history

2.3 The disease starts in the milk-producing cells in the breast, and in the cells lining the small milk-ducts. There is a pre-invasive stage of the cancer during which malignant cells are confined within the duct system. This is followed by an invasive phase when the cancer invades the surrounding tissues and has the potential for spread to local lymph nodes and to distant sites such as the bones, liver and brain. These secondary deposits are called metastases. Although breast cancer may disseminate early in its natural history the rate of growth is variable and in many women it will be several years from the development of the disease

11

to the appearance of metastases in other sites. The main aim of screening is to detect cancers that are still localised to the breast and before secondary spread has occurred.

Recognisable early stage

2.4 It has been shown that up to 20 per cent of the cancers that are too small to be clinically evident are not invasive. Further, invasive cancers that are detected while small (under 1cm in diameter) are less likely to have metastasised to local lymph nodes or distant sites than are larger tumours. These non-invasive and small invasive tumours are generally regarded as constituting 'early stage disease'.

Benefit of treatment at early stage

2.5 It is not enough to compare the survival of patients with screen-detected cancers with the survival of those who present with symptoms. Although a longer survival of patients with screen-detected cancers might be observed, this alone is insufficient evidence that screening has prolonged survival because of various biases that may appear to enhance survival even if screening did not have any effect.

2.6 Firstly, survival is measured from the time of diagnosis, but screening advances the date at which diagnosis is made, thus automatically lengthening the survival time even if it makes no difference to the date of death. This is known as 'lead-time bias'.

2.7 Secondly, fast-growing cancers spend a relatively short time in the phase when they are detectable by screening and are not yet evident to the woman herself. Hence screening is likely to pick up relatively few of these fast-growing cancers and proportionally more of slow-growing or even non-progressive, non-invasive cancers; women with these cancers will anyway have a better survival. This is known as 'length bias'.

2.8 Thirdly, women who take up the offer of screening are likely to be health-aware women who perhaps have a better prognosis anyway than the more fatalistic women who do not accept screening. This is known as 'selection bias'.

2.9 These biases, which may distort survival rates of women whose cancers are detected by screening, can be overcome only by comparing the impact of screening on the number of women who die from breast cancer in a whole population for whom screening is available with a population not offered screening. The randomised trials conducted in New York and Sweden have used this method so that the results reported are free of bias. These results have demonstrated a significant reduction in mortality in those offered screening. Support for these results has come from the case-control studies in the Netherlands which have demonstrated that women who have been screened have a reduced incidence of death from breast cancer compared with those not screened (see Chapter 1 and Annex C).

A suitable screening test: sensitivity and specificity

2.10 Inherent in the definition of screening is the assumption that the screening test does not reach an absolute conclusion on the presence or absence of disease but merely sorts the screened people into test-positives and test-negatives. Test-positive subjects then need to undergo diagnostic tests to find out whether or not they do have breast cancer. A suitable screening test for breast cancer must be able to sort out these two groups as accurately as possible. It must be capable of detecting the great majority of breast cancers present among the screened group (high sensitivity) and give very few false negative results. It must also eliminate from further diagnostic tests the majority of women who do not have breast cancer (high specificity) giving very few false positive results. The table below compares the result of the screening test with the true diagnosis.

Table 2.1 Sensitivity and specificity of screening test for breast cancer

		True Diagnosis	
		Breast Cancer Present	Breast Cancer Absent
Test result	Positive	True Positive (a)	False positive (c)
	Negative	False negative (b)	True negative (d)

Sensitivity is the number of true positives as a proportion of all those with breast cancer present

ie. $\dfrac{(a)}{(a)+(b)}$

Specificity is the number of true negatives as a proportion of all those with breast cancer absent

ie. $\dfrac{(d)}{(c)+(d)}$

2.11 Sensitivity and specificity are inversely related. To achieve a high sensitivity the 'index of suspicion' must be set low so that all the cancers will be classified as positive; but this has the unwanted effect of increasing the number of false positives and hence decreasing specificity. Conversely, in order to achieve a high specificity the 'index of suspicion' for classifying a positive must be high; but this may result in missing a few potentially detectable cancers and hence decreasing sensitivity.

2.12 A problem arises in defining the true incidence of false negative tests for breast cancer because all the women with negative screening tests cannot be subjected to further diagnostic investigation. A convention is to classify as false negatives any cancers that present with symptoms in a 12-month interval after a negative screening test. Some of these so-called 'interval cancers' may have been present in detectable form at the time of screening but were missed by the test, while others may have been fast-growing cancers that were not present at the time of screening and progressed to a detectable phase within 12 months. Either way they represent the cancers that were not picked up by the screening test. This is not an absolute measure of sensitivity; if the intervals were longer than 12 months the sensitivity would be lower.

2.13 The sensitivity and specificity of the various tests used to screen for breast cancer are discussed in detail in Chapter 4.

Acceptability of screening

2.14 Experience in the UK trial indicates that at least 64 per cent of women aged 45–64 will accept a personal invitation from their general practitioner to attend for a first screen. Acceptability drops off with increasing age. It has been shown to be possible to maintain attendance at repeat routine screens at above 60 per cent of the target population. We believe that it should be possible to increase this to 70 per cent. This level of acceptability, while not ideal, was shown in the HIP (New York) study to be sufficient to enable a screening programme to have an impact on breast cancer mortality.

Adequate facilities for diagnosis and treatment of screen-detected abnormalities

2.15 It is important that women with positive test results are thoroughly assessed as quickly as possible. The diagnostic skills required for the assessment of an abnormality include expert clinical examination, sophisticated mammography, fine needle aspiration to discriminate solid from cystic lesions and fine needle aspiration cytology to define the nature of solid lesions. For those women who are still suspected of having cancer after one or more of these tests, biopsy and histological assessment are necessary. If the abnormality is not palpable, particular radiological, surgical and pathological skills are required to ensure correct diagnosis. At present these diagnostic skills are available only in some centres in the UK. The requirements for assessment, biopsy and treatment of screen-detected breast cancers are described in Chapter 6.

Repeated screening

2.16 Since the probability of developing a breast cancer increases with age, screening needs to be repeated at regular intervals. The optimum interval between repeated screens is not known (see Chapter 5).

Physical and psychological harm

2.17 The potential hazards of screening are firstly, that the ionising radiation used in mammography might itself induce some breast cancers; secondly, that unnecessary biopsy operations are performed in women with false positive results; and thirdly, that women might undergo unnecessary procedures for the diagnosis and treatment of cancer which might not have entered an invasive phase during their lifetime. In addition there are psychological consequences which must be considered.

2.18 The evidence on the radiation risk of mammography is reviewed in Annex D. In summary, it suggests that among two million women above the age of 50 receiving a mean dose of radiation of 0.15 cGy to the breast (a dose at the upper end of the range received from screening) one extra breast cancer might develop each year after a latent interval of 10 years. This is less than one thousandth the incidence of naturally occurring breast cancer in women over 50 years old. The radiation risk of regular mammography for screening women over 50 years old is thus insignificant compared with its potential benefits.

2.19 If screening were detecting breast cancers that would otherwise not have been diagnosed, it would be expected that in controlled trials there would be a persistent excess number of breast cancers in the screened group compared with the control group. In the HIP (New York) trial the number of breast cancers diagnosed in the two groups was equal after 7 years. Over-diagnosis was not a problem. It is possible that with the improvement in sensitivity of mammography that has since occurred, over-diagnosis may happen, and after 6 years in the Two Counties (Sweden) trial 20 per cent more cancers have been diagnosed in the group offered screening compared with those presenting in the control group. Further follow-up is required to find out whether this excess persists for the life-span of the women.

2.20 Concern has been expressed that screening may provoke anxiety about breast cancer in some women. However, psychological studies comparing women attending a screening clinic with other women of the same age have not revealed any excess in anxiety or depression that might require psychiatric treatment in the screened group. Among women who are found to have a positive test anxiety is naturally a problem, and the severity of this is currently under investigation.

Balance between benefit and cost

2.21 Because of the difficulty of defining health benefits in monetary terms, a cost-utility analysis has been used to assess breast cancer screening in terms of the cost per extra year of life gained. The results of the analysis can then be compared with the cost per life-year gained of other health service activities. An economic appraisal of breast cancer screening is presented in Chapter 9.

Figure 3.1   Screening Procedure

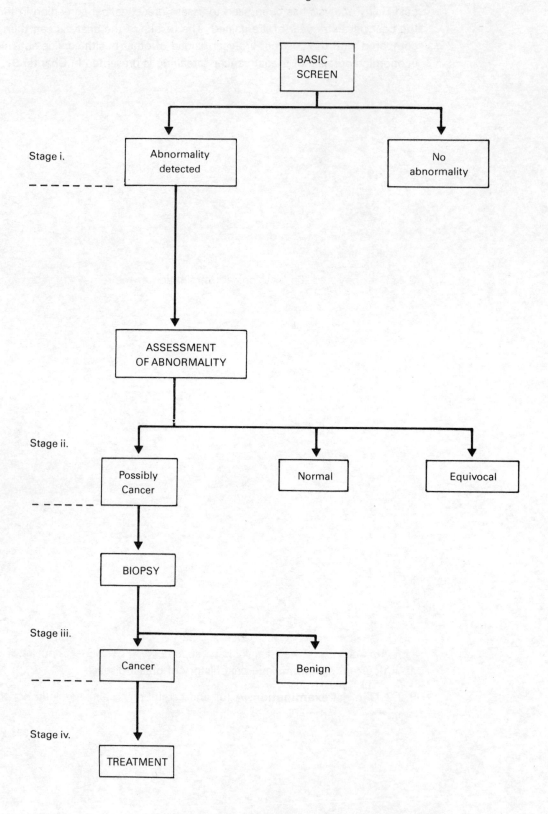

Notes: a) If the basic screen is single-view mammography stage i may
          include additional mammographic views.

       b) Women with equivocal assessment results are kept under
          surveillance by the assessment team.

       c) Normal at stage ii includes benign lesions considered
          insignificant.

3 Screening procedure

3.1 The screening procedure may be divided into the following four stages:

3.1.1 **the basic screen** to detect an abnormality which may or may not be cancer;

3.1.2 **the assessment** of the abnormality to determine whether a surgical biopsy is required;

3.1.3 **biopsy** and the histological examination of the removed tissue; and

3.1.4 **treatment** of screen-detected cancers.

A flow diagram is shown in Figure 3.1 opposite.

Stage i. The basic screen

3.2 A number of different methods have been suggested as a basic screening test to detect asymptomatic breast cancer. Below are the three methods that have been used separately or in combination in breast cancer screening trials.

3.2.1 **Mammography.** An X-ray technique which has been specially developed for taking images of the breast. Mammography can detect tumours that cannot be detected by a clinical examination. Radiographers, using specially designed equipment, take one or more X-ray views of each breast. The woman is positioned so that the entire breast tissue is included on the film (mammogram). The films, which must be of high quality, are usually read in batches after the screening session by either radiologists, other doctors (eg clinical medical officers) or other health professionals (eg radiographers). A single medio-lateral oblique view may be taken at the initial visit with, if necessary, recall for a repeat oblique and cranio-caudal view at a subsequent visit. Alternatively, these two views may both be taken at the initial visit. When mammography has been the only method used it has usually been accompanied by a questionnaire or enquiry about current symptoms and past history of breast disease.

3.2.2 **Clinical examination.** A full and careful physical examination of the breast by trained medical or nursing personnel.

3.2.3 **Breast self-examination (BSE).** The regular examination (eg monthly) of the breast by the woman herself. She may be instructed by medical or other health professionals to detect visible abnormalities (eg skin dimpling, discrete lumps and asymmetry) and palpable lumps. Instruction may also be available through the media, leaflets or videos.

3.3 Other suggested techniques include thermography, ultrasonography, telediaphonography, computed tomography and magnetic resonance imaging. In addition to these imaging techniques there is the cytological examination of cells aspirated from the nipple. However, at the present, only mammography, clinical examination and BSE warrant further examination for use in mass population screening. These options are evaluated in Chapter 4.

Figure 3.2

Flow chart illustrating possible options for referral of women with definite or possible abnormalities found at basic screening.

Routes for notification only are not shown.

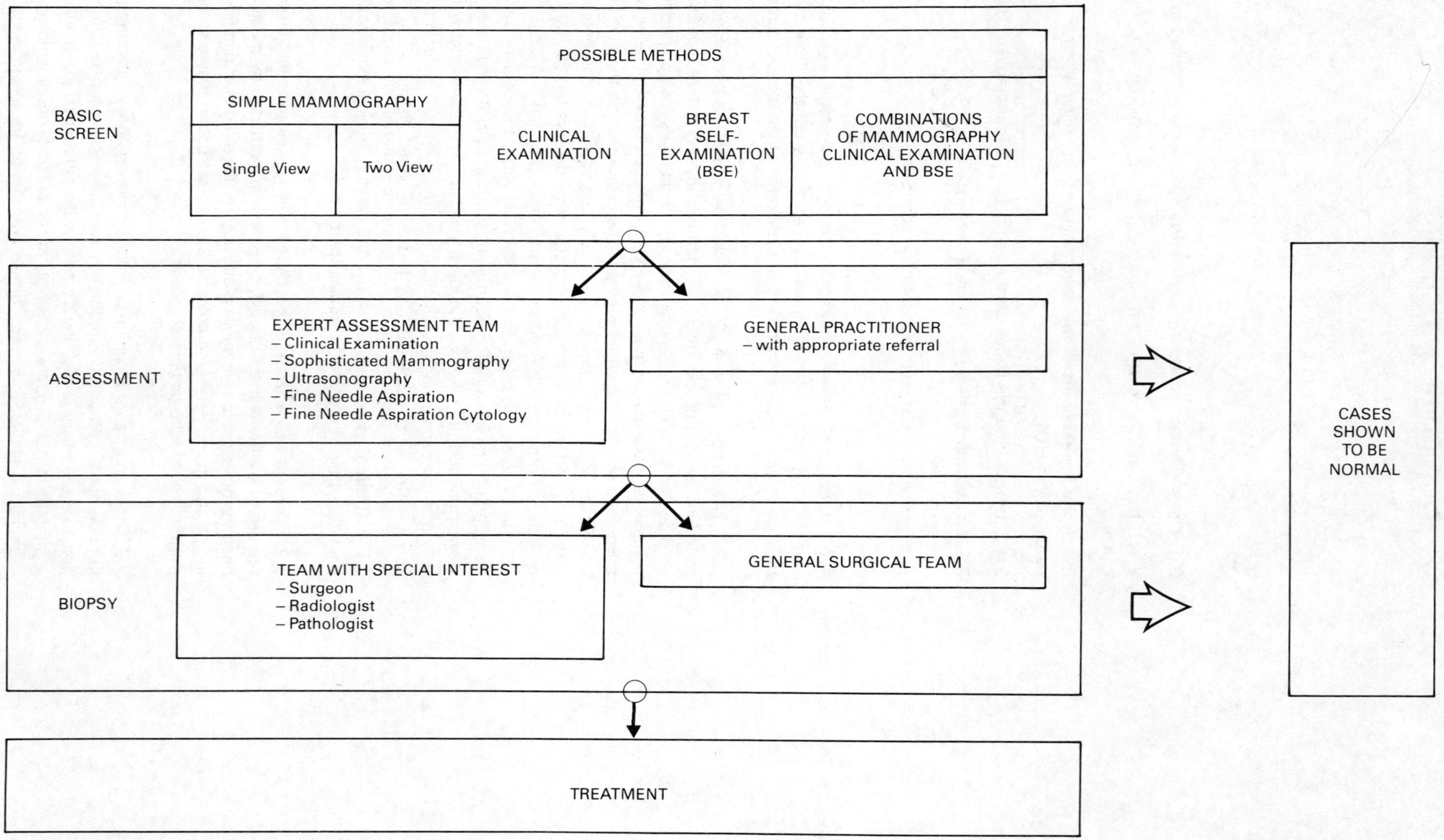

BASIC SCREEN

POSSIBLE METHODS

SIMPLE MAMMOGRAPHY
- Single View
- Two View

CLINICAL EXAMINATION

BREAST SELF-EXAMINATION (BSE)

COMBINATIONS OF MAMMOGRAPHY CLINICAL EXAMINATION AND BSE

ASSESSMENT

EXPERT ASSESSMENT TEAM
- Clinical Examination
- Sophisticated Mammography
- Ultrasonography
- Fine Needle Aspiration
- Fine Needle Aspiration Cytology

GENERAL PRACTITIONER
- with appropriate referral

BIOPSY

TEAM WITH SPECIAL INTEREST
- Surgeon
- Radiologist
- Pathologist

GENERAL SURGICAL TEAM

TREATMENT

CASES SHOWN TO BE NORMAL

Stage ii. Assessment

3.4 Basic screening methods identify abnormalities or suspicious lesions which are often impalpable ie not clinically apparent as a breast lump. These methods cannot by themselves diagnose breast cancer. The definitive diagnosis of breast cancer requires histological examination of a biopsy specimen. It would be impracticable, expensive and would make screening less acceptable if all women with abnormal results had a surgical biopsy. In addition a surgical biopsy is not without risk, may cause the woman distress, and leaves a scar which may make subsequent basic screening tests more difficult to interpret.

3.5 Evidence from the Two Counties (Sweden) trial shows that for every 1,000 women who were screened 52 or 5 per cent of the women had a suspected abnormality detected by mammography but only 6 were later found to have breast cancer. Similar figures have been found in the UK trials except for the initial prevalence screen when 8 per cent – 10 per cent of screened women were suspected of having an abnormality.

3.6 To keep the number of biopsies down to an acceptable level requires expert assessment of screen-detected abnormalities. A range of techniques is available for assessment (see Chapter 6). These techniques can most effectively be carried out by a multidisciplinary team including a clinical examiner, radiologist and pathologist, all with a special interest in breast cancer and experience of the techniques used for its diagnosis.

3.7 Figure 3.2 (opposite) shows two referral routes by which a woman with a screen-detected abnormality could be assessed. In one, the general practitioner, upon receipt of a report, takes responsibility and may refer the woman for such specialist advice as he or she considers necessary. This could be to an individual specialist of their choice at a surgical outpatients or, if available, to a specialist assessment team. In the other route, the woman would be referred from the basic screening team, with the prior consent of the general practitioner, to a specialist assessment team.

Stage iii. Biopsy

3.8 An open or excision biopsy is a surgical procedure by which a suspected lesion is removed from the breast for histological examination. This would be performed by a surgeon who may be a member of a specialist breast team. The pattern of referral depends on availability, the wishes of the general practitioner and the woman herself. Patients could also be referred to a specialist surgeon from the assessment team; conversely a specialist surgeon may be an active member of that team. The biopsy of impalpable abnormalities requires special radiological and surgical localisation techniques and skilled pathology.

Stage iv. Treatment

3.9 Treatment of screen-detected cancers is the last stage in the screening procedure. In view of the complex methods now available this is increasingly being undertaken by a team with a special interest in breast cancer, supported by suitably trained nurses and other health professionals.

3.10 The facilities required for the assessment, biopsy and treatment of screen-detected abnormalities are considered further in Chapter 6.

Table 4.1 Summarised Evidence on Sensitivity, Specificity and Acceptability of Screening Tests

Centre	Start of trial	Age range	Method	Sensitivity		Specificity		Acceptability	
				Initial round	Subsequent round	Initial round	Subsequent round	Initial round	Subsequent round
Health Insurance Plan (HIP) (New York)	1963	40–64	CM_2	81%	69%	–	–	66%	–
Breast Cancer Detection Demonstration Projects (BCDDP) (USA)	1973	35–	CM_2	85%	77%	95%	97%	–	–
Manchester	1973	40–	CM_2	–	–	93%	94%	–	–
West London	1973	40–	CM_2	96%	60%	87%	96%	–	–
Utrecht (Netherlands)	1975	50–64	CM_2	96%	91%	96%	99%	72%	58%
Nijmegen (Netherlands)	1975	33–	M_1	–	87% (3 rounds)	–	99% (3 rounds)	85%	65%
Ostergötland and Kopparberg County (Sweden)	1977	40–74	M_1	96%	–	96%	97%	89%	–
Malmö (Sweden)	1966	16–67	C	47%	50%	94%	94%	81%	–
Malmö (Sweden)	1977	45–69	M_2	78%	77%	97%	97%	73%	70%
Gävle (Sweden)	1974	35–	M_1	94%	–	–	–	88%	–
Edinburgh	1979	45–64	CM_1 or CM_2	91%	90%	97%	99%	64%	–
Edinburgh	1979	45–64	C	–	78%	–	97%	–	55%
Guildford	1979	45–64	CM_1	94%	86%	92%	95%	69%	64%
Guildford	1979	45–64	C	–	58%	–	92%	–	63%
Huddersfield	1979	45–64	BSE	–	–	–	–	31%	–
Nottingham	1979	45–64	BSE	–	–	–	–	52%	–

Key
C = Clinical examination
M_1 = Single-view mammography
M_2 = Two-view mammography
BSE = Breast Self-Examination

Notes

1. Sensitivity = $$\frac{\text{Number of screen-detected cancers} \times 100}{\text{Number of screen-detected cancers} + \text{Number of cancers detected in following 12 months}}$$

2. Specificity = $$\frac{\text{Number of women found negative at the basic screen} \times 100}{\text{Number of women without cancer}}$$

3. Acceptance in subsequent round equals women attending at least one other round as a percentage of those in the target population
4. BCDDP: Mammography for those under 50 years ceased from 1977
5. West London: Sensitivity for initial round was measured after 6 months
6. Malmö: M_2 to M_1 from 3rd screening for lower density breasts
7. Edinburgh: Changed from M_1 to M_2
8. Huddersfield and Nottingham: Acceptability refers to attendance at a BSE teaching session

4 Basic screening methods

Introduction

4.1 The decision about which screening method to use must rest upon evidence of the ability of each method to detect a high proportion of asymptomatic cancers at a stage when prognosis can be improved by treatment, and this in turn depends upon how acceptable each method is to women and upon its sensitivity (see Chapter 2). The disadvantages of a method in terms of lack of specificity (leading to further investigation of many women without cancer) and cost are also relevant.

4.2 In the previous chapter various methods for basic screening were described. Mammography, clinical examination and breast self-examination (BSE), used separately or in combination, appeared to be the only methods that warrant further examination for use in mass population screening. In this chapter we assess the effectiveness, acceptability, sensitivity, specificity, and unit cost of each of these methods. Details of unit costs for the basic screen and assessment stages are at Annex E. Results from various studies are set out in Table 4.1 opposite. These results have to be used with caution because the studies have been carried out at different times and under different conditions. Below each method is assessed first when used as the sole screening method and then when used in combination.

4.3 Mammography

4.3.1 **Effectiveness.** Studies that have used mammography as the sole screening method – Two Counties (Sweden) and Nijmegen (Netherlands) – provide evidence that mammography alone is effective in reducing mortality (See Annex C).

4.3.2 **Acceptability** In the Two Counties (Sweden) study women were recruited for mammography screening by personal invitation and acceptance rates of up to 90 per cent were obtained. From present experience we expect that acceptance rates in the UK would be about 70 per cent.

4.3.3 **Sensitivity.** Modern high-quality mammography can be a very sensitive test; in some Swedish studies single-view mammography has detected over 90 per cent of breast cancers (the remaining 10 per cent or less being interval cancers diagnosed within 12 months of a negative screening test). Other European studies using single or two-view mammographic screening have reported lower sensititivities of around 80 per cent. Differences between results may be due to differences in the quality of mammograms and their interpretation.

4.3.4 **Specificity.** The specificity of mammography is influenced by quality of mammograms and is also dependent on the expertise and experience of the personnel who read them. The specificity of mammography in the initial screen in some reported overseas studies is 95 per cent or more. Routine screens in subsequent years tend to have a higher specificity. Neither the relative sensitivities nor relative specificities of single versus two-view mammography in screening have been adequately studied.

4.3.5 Cost. The Two Counties (Sweden) study has costed the use of mammography as a sole basic screening method at £10–£11 per woman (1983–84 prices). In the Edinburgh study in which mammography is used with clinical examination the cost of the mammography component has been estimated for single-view at £11.66 and for two-view at £15.03 (1983–84 prices). These costs include the cost of assessment.

4.3.6 Conclusion. Mammography used as a sole screening method is highly effective, acceptable, sensitive, specific and has a reasonable cost.

4.4 Clinical Examination

4.4.1 Effectiveness. The effectiveness of clinical examination used alone in reducing mortality from breast cancer has not been tested. One trial in progress in Canada is comparing breast cancer mortality among women aged 50 to 59 who are screened by clinical examination with those screened by both clinical examination and mammography (see Annex C). However since there is no unscreened control group, this trial will not be able to quantify the effectiveness of clinical examination alone.

4.4.2 Acceptability. The level of acceptance of invitations to attend for initial screening by clinical examination is unknown but is likely to be similar to that for mammography. In the UK trials information is available on attendance for clinical examination on its own only among those women who had attended a previous screening round, which included mammography. Ninety per cent of those who had attended previously accepted the invitation for clinical screening.

4.4.3 Sensitivity. In one early Swedish study in Malmö using clinical examination alone sensitivity was only 47 per cent. In Edinburgh a sensitivity of 78 per cent has been obtained, whereas in Guildford it has been 58 per cent.

4.4.4 Specificity. In the early Swedish study in Malmö specificity was 94 per cent. In one early UK study among self-selected women, clinical examination had a low specificity of 92 per cent, and the same has been found more recently in Guildford. In the Edinburgh study it was 97 per cent.

4.4.5 Cost. In the Edinburgh study the cost of performing a clinical examination, including the cost of assessment, is estimated at £5.94 (1983–84 prices).

4.4.6 Conclusion. There is no evidence that clinical examination is effective in reducing mortality from breast cancer. It has a lower sensitivity than mammography.

4.5 Breast self-examination (BSE)

4.5.1 Effectiveness. There is no clear evidence that BSE reduces breast cancer mortality. Two trials in progress will test the effectiveness of particular policies of educating women to perform BSE. One is the multicentre UK trial in which mortality in two health districts, where every woman aged 45–64 has been invited to a BSE class, is being compared with that in two screening districts and four control districts. Another trial of BSE education in factories and polyclinics is starting in the USSR. If results of those studies are negative this will not necessarily mean that BSE itself is not effective; it could be that the educational policy failed to persuade sufficient women to perform it correctly. There is some evidence that BSE contributes to a reduction in tumour size at diagnosis. This is supported by preliminary findings of BSE education trials and by studies employing theoretical computer models.

4.5.2 Acceptability. Failure to practise BSE seems to be a major disadvantage to the use of BSE as a sole screening method. In a mass programme in one district in the UK trial only a third, and in the other, half of the invited women attended a BSE class. Interview surveys have found that even without an education programme about one quarter of women aged 45 to 64 say that they are already practising some form of BSE. Following class attendance this may increase to about one half.

4.5.3 **Sensitivity.** This is impossible to measure in a way comparable to that used for other screening tests – ie based on cancers arising within a stated interval after a negative examination. However, one of the assumptions underlying BSE is that the frequency with which a woman may examine her own breasts enables her to detect an abnormality earlier than could less frequent clinical examinations by health professionals.

4.5.4 **Specificity.** Various surveys suggest that BSE education campaigns have not been accompanied by a major increase in medical consultations nor in breast biopsies. In the two BSE districts in the UK trial only about 1 per cent of the target population of women aged 45–64 attend self-referral diagnostic breast clinics each year but the proportion who attend their general practitioner is unknown. Thus, although an exact figure cannot be put on the number of false positive results of BSE, it is likely that its specificity is high, at least in women aged over 45. In younger women (among whom minor benign breast disease is more common and malignant disease much less common) the specificity of BSE is lower.

4.5.5 **Cost.** In the UK trial the cost of BSE education involving group teaching is £2.57–£11.44 (1983–84 prices) per woman taught. (The wide range reflects different attendance rates). Teaching on an individual basis would be more expensive.

4.5.6 **Conclusion.** There is no evidence to show that BSE is effective in reducing mortality from breast cancer. It is not as sensitive as mammography in detecting small tumours and has a low specificity in younger women. Lack of evidence on its effectiveness should not, however, discourage women from practising BSE. It is reasonable to assume that it contributes to earlier diagnosis.

4.6 Combinations of clinical examination, mammography and BSE

Most of the past studies of screening have used a combination of clinical examination and mammography. Some have also included education in BSE.

4.6.1 **Effectiveness.** Both the (HIP) New York study and the Utrecht (Netherlands) study have shown that screening combining clinical examination and mammography can reduce mortality. It is not possible to quantify how much of the benefit was achieved by using the combined methods as opposed to either on its own. A Canadian study (see paragraph 4.4.1) will compare the effectiveness of clinical examination plus mammography with that of clinical examination alone.

4.6.2 **Acceptability.** There appears to be little, if any, difference between the acceptability of combined-method screening and single-method screening. Acceptance of BSE when it is individually taught in association with clinical examination or mammography may be greater than when it is taught in groups or by media. This also is being studied in the Canadian trials.

4.6.3 **Sensitivity.** Sensitivity of both methods combined is 94 per cent in Guildford and 91 per cent in Edinburgh: this is in line with other studies.

4.6.4 **Specificity.** The specificity of combined clinical and mammographic screening is about 95 per cent at first screening and slightly more at subsequent screenings.

4.6.5 Cost. The addition of extra methods may add to the cost not only of basic screening but also of further assessment. In the Edinburgh study the cost of a combined mammographic and clinical screen, including the cost of the assessment, is £12.86 (single-view mammography) and £16.23 (two-view mammography) (1983–84 prices). The addition of individual B S E education would increase costs if it led to a reduction in the number of women who could be screened per session.

Discussion

4.7 On the information currently available, mammography alone is the preferred option for basic screening. Unlike clinical examination and B S E used alone it is of proven effectiveness in reducing breast cancer mortality among women aged 50 and over. Clinical examination and B S E detect fewer of the early tumours for which treatment may have the most effect on survival. Mammography is acceptable to women. Its sensitivity is considerably greater than that of clinical examination and its specificity in recalling women for further investigation is also high. Any carcinogenic risk arising from its radiation is minute in relation to its potential benefits in women aged 50 and over. It carries a potential disadvantage of detecting early lesions that may never prove life-threatening and would not normally present for treatment but this is mainly limited to the initial prevalence screen, and is of less importance in subsequent screens.

4.8. Any benefit resulting from combined as opposed to single-method screening must arise from the extra sensitivity gained by using two (or more) tests as opposed to one. This is difficult to assess. Twenty years ago, in the (HIP) New York study 42 per cent of screen-detected cases would have been missed if only mammography had been used and 33 per cent if only clinical examination had been used. Since then mammographic techniques have improved substantially so that in current studies using both clinical examination and mammography only 5–10 per cent of cases would be missed if only mammography were used. However, the objective of screening is not case-detection but improved prognosis for cases detected at screening. The marginal cost of adding clinical examination to mammography is high in terms of cancers detected (see Annex E) but is unknown in terms of life-years gained.

4.9. The extent of any gain from including B S E education in the screening procedure is also difficult to assess because the method of assessing sensitivity assumes that any cancers diagnosed in the 12 months following a screen are "false negatives" to that screen. However, these cases may be "true positives" to the B S E-education component of combined-method screening because the woman has detected them herself earlier than if she had not been encouraged to perform B S E. Hence a screening programme incorporating B S E education may appear to have a higher number of interval cases because it increases the number of cancers detected by the woman herself. This programme will appear to have a low sensitivity but it may still achieve a higher proportion of cancers diagnosed at an early stage – and a greater reduction in mortality – than programmes without B S E education. The additional benefit to be gained by adding B S E education to mammography would probably be greater the longer the interval between mammographic screens.

Conclusions

4.10 High-quality single medio-lateral oblique view mammography has been shown to be an effective method in reducing mortality from breast cancer and we conclude that initially this is the preferred option for the development of mass population screening.

4.11 There is no evidence that clinical examination or breast self-examination is effective when used alone. These methods have some value when used in combination with mammography but their contribution requires further assessment.

4.12 The remainder of our report assumes that single-view mammography is the method to be employed for basic screening in a mass population screening programme.

5 Basic screening, selection and frequency

Introduction

5.1 For any screening programme to achieve maximum efficiency it should be concentrated on those members of the population most likely to benefit from it. In the case of breast cancer this means those women who are most likely to develop breast disease and in whom the prognosis can be altered by screening.

Selection by age

5.2 The most important risk factor for breast cancer is age. Figure B−2 at Annex B shows how the incidence and mortality rates increase with age so that for women aged 50−54 incidence is over seven times and mortality is over twelve times that of women aged 30−34.

5.3 Screening policy should ideally be based not merely on the age groups most likely to develop breast cancer, but on those in whom early detection can improve the prognosis. All of the studies that have so far examined the effect of screening on deaths from breast cancer have clearly shown its value for women aged 50 and over but at younger ages its effectiveness is less and is uncertain.

5.4 The information from these studies is difficult to interpret because screening clearly influences the age at diagnosis (cases being diagnosed at younger ages than if they were left unscreened). Age-specific effects are, therefore, analysed according to the age at which a woman enters the study ie the age at which she was first invited to be screened. In the Two Counties (Sweden) and Nijmegen (Netherlands) studies no difference in the breast cancer mortality rate between study and control groups has been reported among women aged less than 50 at entry. The same finding applied in the early reports from HIP (New York) study but the longer-term follow-up which is now available has revealed a difference in favour of the study group. In women aged 45−49 a lower mortality from breast cancer in the study group began to appear 6 years after their entry to the trial (when they were aged 51−55), and in those aged 40−44 at entry a more modest effect only became apparent at the 9th year of follow-up (when they were aged 49−53). Statistical tests indicate that these differences could have occurred by chance but it is important that these results are kept under review.

5.5 Additional evidence on the effect of screening women of different ages comes from estimates of the lead-time gained by screening (ie the interval between the date of detection by screening and the date when symptomatic diagnosis would have occurred if the woman had not been screened). In the HIP (New York) study for women aged under 50 the average lead-time gained by screening was less than 6 months, compared with nearly 2 years in women aged 50−59 at entry. It would be expected that improvements in mammography since the HIP (New York) study would result in longer average lead-times among women aged under 50 in more recent trials.

5.6 The benefit of screening women aged 65 and over is also open to question, but for different reasons. One is the lower acceptance of screening by women at older ages. In the Utrecht (Netherlands) study there was a rapid fall off in acceptance of repeated screening over age 65 which has also been observed in the UK trial. In the Two Counties (Sweden) study a reduction in breast cancer mortality has been reported up to the age of 74, but acceptance rates in this study are over 80 per cent even up to this age. Another reason for lower benefit in older women is their increasing chance of dying of diseases other than breast cancer. Finally, breast cancer diagnosed in older women appears to run a less aggressive course than when diagnosed in younger women.

5.7 **Conclusion.** There is clear evidence that women aged 50 and over are likely to benefit from screening. Further evidence on the effectiveness of screening women under 50 is required: studies are continuing in the UK, Canada and Sweden. Women up to age 65 should be positively encouraged to be regularly screened, but after this age screening should be provided only for those who request it.

Selection by other risk factors

5.8 As well as age a number of other factors are known that identify a woman as being at increased risk of breast cancer. Many of these are associated with reproductive function, probably indicating the influence of female sex hormones on the development of breast cancer. These factors include early menarche, late menopause and late age at first full-term pregnancy. Other risk factors include a family history of breast cancer, particularly in mothers or sisters; and a history of benign breast disease. It should be noted that although these risk factors have been identified the cause of breast cancer is still unknown.

5.9 The excess risk conferred by each of these factors separately is not very great — less than two-fold. If used in combination to identify high risk women (eg a woman whose mother has had breast cancer, who has had her first baby at age 35 and who has a history of atypical change in the breast epithelium) the prediction of risk is much greater. But there are so few such women among the general population that provision of screening for them but not for others would have a negligible impact on breast cancer mortality.

5.10 The use of tests to 'pre-screen' women and select out a high risk group for regular routine screening has been investigated. These pre-screening tests include measuring the levels of circulating hormones and examining mammographic patterns of breast structure. So far none of these tests is sufficiently sensitive to select a minority of women in whom the majority of breast cancers will occur. It is hoped that further research will identify measurements more specific to breast cancer.

5.11 **Conclusion.** The use of risk factors other than age to identify women in the general population who should be screened is not practicable at present. This is not to say that individual patients who have sought advice about breast problems and who have one or more recognised risk factors should not be investigated, but it is for the responsible clinician to decide. For a population screening programme the only feasible criterion for selection at present is initially to limit screening to women aged 50 and over.

Frequency

5.12 As the probability of developing breast cancer increases with age, a single negative screen does not mean that a woman has lifetime protection against the disease. Screening therefore needs to be repeated at intervals.

5.13 For screening to detect all cancers it would be necessary to screen more frequently than the time taken for the fastest growing cancer to progress from being undetectable to presenting with symptoms. But the rate of growth of the disease is very variable with some cancers probably passing through this phase in days or weeks while others may take years or even decades.

5.14 In practice decisions on the interval between routine repeat screens are inevitably compromises, aiming to let as few cancers as possible escape detection by screening while at the same time aiming to minimise the costs and disadvantages of screening too frequently. Value judgements about the relative costs of missing a case or of screening 'too often' have been the basis for the arbitrary decisions on rescreening intervals in most studies and very little research has been done on this subject.

5.15 Many trials including the HIP (New York) study, most other American work, and the current UK Trials have chosen a 1-year interval between screens. There is probably a general agreement that rescreening more frequently than yearly is not really feasible. The Two Counties (Sweden) and Netherlands studies have used intervals longer than a year. In Nijmegen, the interval between repeat screens was 2 years. In the Two Counties (Sweden) study the average screening interval was 33 months for women aged 50 and over and 22 months for women aged 40 to 49. In Utrecht, the first cohort of women to be enrolled were rescreened at intervals of 12 months, then 18 months, then 24 months, then 48 months. As expected these studies have shown that the longer the interval the more cancers arise during it.

5.16 In the Swedish Two Counties study it has been found that among women aged 50–69 screening detects 86 per cent of the cancers expected to arise in the following year, 70 per cent of those expected in the next (2nd) year and 54 per cent of those expected in the next 6 months. Overall, 74 per cent of the expected incidence over the 30-months period was detected by screening.

5.17 By implication, with increasing intervals there is a fall in the protection against cancer mortality conferred by screening, but this has not been quantified. It might be postulated that cases presenting in the intervals between screens would be fast-growing cancers with a relatively poor prognosis, but in the HIP (New York) and the Two Counties (Sweden) studies comparisons of the survival of these cases with that of all breast cancers diagnosed in the control group has shown no difference between the two. Various forms of mathematical and computer simulation modelling based either on New York data or on assumptions about growth rates and test sensitivities have concluded that different intervals may be appropriate for different ages, with younger women needing a shorter interval than older women.

5.18 **Conclusion.** There is clearly a need for further research into the cost and benefits of screening at different intervals to identify an optimum screening interval. The Swedish study shows a substantial benefit in women aged 50 and over with a screening interval of nearly 3 years. Until the optimum frequency has been determined we suggest that the interval should be 3 years.

Conclusions

5.19 The effectiveness of screening has so far been demonstrated only for women aged 50 and over. In view of the poor response rates there is insufficient benefit to be gained by actively offering screening to women aged 65 and over. The priority of any screening programme should, therefore, be given to offering an initial screen to as many women as possible aged between 50–64 years. This does not exclude making screening available on demand to older women.

5.20 The use of risk factors other than age to identify women in the general population who should be screened is not practicable at present.

5.21 There is insufficient evidence on the optimum frequency for routine repeated screening and its determination must have high priority for immediate research. As a starting point for the screening programme we suggest an interval of 3 years but this must be kept under review.

6 Assessment, biopsy and treatment

Recall for additional films

6.1 In Chapter 4 we concluded that mammography alone was the preferred option for basic screening. We also concluded that high quality single-view mammography could be effective. When only a single-view is used it is estimated that up to 10 per cent of the women screened might be required to have an additional cranio-caudal view and a repeat medio-lateral view to define the nature of an artefact or composite shadow. This would be done at a subsequent visit to the basic screening unit.

Assessment

6.2 When a basic screening result is confirmed as abnormal it must be assessed. In addition any women who report symptoms, eg a breast lump or distortion, at the basic screen must be referred for assessment.

6.3 In Chapter 3 we listed the following techniques which were available for the assessment of screen detected abnormalities:

Clinical examination

Sophisticated mammography

Ultrasonography

Fine needle aspiration

Fine needle aspiration cytology.

6.4 **Clinical Examination.** All women referred for assessment must have a clinical examination of the breast to establish whether palpable lesions are present in the light of mammographic findings. It is essential that this examination is carried out by a clinician experienced in the signs and symptoms of early breast cancer.

6.5 **Sophisticated Mammography.** For suspicious lesions, additional mammographic study is necessary using machines not only with moving grids, but also with facilities for magnification views and needle localisation techniques. These units are more sophisticated than the simpler machines appropriate for basic screening and are therefore more expensive. Such machines are likely to be located in a hospital, where they will also be used for the investigation of symptomatic patients.

6.6 **Ultrasonography.** Ultrasound cannot at present be used as a basic screening technique because it fails to detect the majority of solid impalpable lesions. However, when used to complement mammography it is a valuable assessment technique, eg to confirm the cystic nature of an impalpable lesion or to help in guided-needle biopsy or sampling. A simple machine is considered satisfactory.

6.7 **Fine Needle Aspiration.** This is a valuable method for differentiating cystic from solid lesions. This applies not only to palpable lesions, but also to impalpable small mammographic opacities. For the aspiration of these small lesions ultrasonic guidance is helpful.

6.8 **Fine Needle Aspiration Cytology.** This technique is used to examine cells aspirated from suspicious solid lesions, whether palpable or impalpable. Its place in differentiating benign from malignant lesions is now established.

6.9 It is now considered desirable that all these techniques are available for the assessment of abnormal results suspected from basic screening. Where cytology is not available, excision biopsy would require to be carried out on a larger number of suspicious lesions leading to an increased ratio of benign to malignant biopsies.

6.10 **Specialist assessment teams.** In Chapter 3 we described two possible routes by which a screen-detected abnormality could be referred for assessment. The basic screening unit would refer a woman either to her general practitioner or, with the prior consent of the general practitioner, direct to a specialist assessment team. If the general practitioner chooses to arrange the assessment, he or she may decide to refer the woman to a surgeon of their choice. If the surgeon does not have access to the specialised assessment techniques this may lead to a high biopsy rate together with a higher ratio of benign to malignant biopsies.

6.11 In existing UK trial centres almost all general practitioners have preferred that the screening team refer women with suspected abnormalities directly to a specialist assessment team, in which event the general practitioner must be kept informed. Some general practitioners may wish to be consulted if an excision biopsy is recommended; others are willing to accept the advice of the assessment team.

6.12 The assessment team consists of a clinician, a radiologist and a pathologist all trained in the diagnosis of breast disease, supported by a radiographer, a nurse and a receptionist. The clinician not only has to be responsible for clinically examining the breasts and possibly performing fine needle aspiration, but also has an important role, in consultation with colleagues, in co-ordinating the results of the investigations, and in making a decision as to whether the lesion merits biopsy. The clinician must also discuss the implications with the woman concerned. In centres with a surgeon having a special interest in breast disease it is likely that the surgeon will wish to be associated with the assessment procedure. However the surgeon may have insufficient time to participate actively, and responsibility for co-ordinating the assessment procedure will fall to another clinician who may or may not be a member of the surgeon's team. It is unlikely that the pattern will be the same in each centre. In Edinburgh and Guildford the clinician in charge of the basic screening unit has assumed this role.

6.13 The advantages of an assessment team are as follows:

6.13.1 continued sharing of experience and review of cases within a multidisciplinary team;

6.13.2 immediate co-ordination of clinical, radiological and pathological findings to reach a decision on the need for a biopsy or treatment as soon as possible;

6.13.3 fine needle aspiration under mammographic and ultrasonic control may be done at the first attendance and immediate cytological reporting may be available.

6.14 Hospital or community-based clinic. The assessment techniques may be carried out either in a hospital or in a clinic in the community. The choice will depend on local circumstances, for example population density. If the choice is a hospital, it is desirable that women are seen separately from those attending a diagnostic clinic for symptomatic women.

Biopsy

6.15 An open or excision biopsy may be carried out either under local or general anaesthesia. X-ray localisation techniques are required for the impalpable lesion, removal of which must be confirmed by specimen radiology best carried out using dedicated apparatus. Similarly, the histological examination of these specimens requires radiological as well as histological facilities. We consider there is no place for the examination of these lesions by frozen section technology.

6.16 The ratio of benign to malignant biopsies reflects the quality of assessment of suspicious lesions. In the UK trials the ratio of benign to malignant biopsies, following the first or prevalence screen, is about two-to-one; following subsequent screens, this ratio is reduced to one-to-one.

6.17 An excision biopsy may be performed by a specialist surgical team or by a general surgeon, depending on availability and the wishes of the general practitioner. Recognised advantages of a specialist surgical team include:

6.17.1 more conversant with the diagnostic procedures used;

6.17.2 more likely to remove palpable masses under local rather than general anaesthesia (with saving of in-patient time and facilities);

6.17.3 skilled in the techniques of localisation biopsy of impalpable lesions and therefore less radical and distorting biopsies;

6.17.4 close liaison with the radiologist and pathologist responsible for the localisation and examination of small lesions;

6.17.5 experience of the various treatment options for small cancers and of the existence of protocols of management either within or apart from controlled therapeutic trials;

6.17.6 more likely to be aware of women's anxieties about breast biopsy and to have specialised nurses to inform and support the women.

Treatment

6.18 Screening is not likely to lead to a significant increase in the numbers of breast cancers treated. During the initial (prevalence) screen there will be an increase in the numbers treated, but this may eventually be compensated by a subsequent reduction in the normally expected incidence. The only potential source of a general increase in the numbers treated would seem to be from cancers that would not otherwise be detected because death from another cause may occur prior to any symptoms arising. The detection of a larger number of *in situ* cancers and small invasive cancers will favour the use of conservation techniques and this may increase certain aspects of therapeutic workload; for example, radiotherapy.

Conclusions

6.19 The assessment of screen-detected abnormalities requires specialised techniques. These techniques are best carried out by a skilled multidisciplinary team, either within a hospital or in a clinic in the community. This team should consist of a clinician, a radiologist and a

pathologist all trained in the diagnosis of breast disease, supported by a radiographer, a nurse and a receptionist. The availability of such teams is an essential prerequisite of a screening service for breast cancer.

6.20 Biopsies of impalpable screen-detected abnormalities should be performed, wherever possible, by a specialist breast team experienced in the surgical, radiological and pathological skills necessary for localisation techniques.

6.21 During the prevalence screen there will be an increase in the numbers to be biopsied and treated for breast cancer. While this may initially increase workload there should be a subsequent reduction to the normally expected incidence. The detection of a larger number of *in situ* cancers and small invasive cancers will favour the use of conservation techniques and this may increase certain aspects of therapeutic workload; for example, radiotherapy.

7 Organisation of a screening service

Introduction

7.1 The evidence reviewed in previous chapters leads us to conclude that a screening service for women aged 50 to 64 using mammography for the basic screen is initially the preferred option. Although evidence on the best interval between repeat screens is still unclear we suggested in Chapter 5 that a 3-year interval may be used during the development of a screening programme but that research is required to determine the optimum interval. This chapter suggests how such a screening service may be organised in the United Kingdom, and is based on the experience of the Edinburgh and Guildford screening programmes which form part of the UK Trial of Early Detection of Breast Cancer. It is only an illustration of how a screening programme may be organised; we accept that other arrangements may be preferred in the light of local circumstances.

7.2 In paragraphs 7.3–7.14 we describe the organisation of the screening process from a woman's entry to the programme, through the basic screening stage, to the follow-up of positive basic screening tests. We describe the organisation of a screening record system in paragraphs 7.15–7.19. Quality control of mammography, radiation protection and monitoring, and the management of a screening service are discussed in paragraphs 7.20–7.24.

Identifying women to be screened

7.3 The eligible population can best be identified from the registers of women on general practitioners' lists. These lists, held by Family Practitioner Committees (FPC) in England and Wales and by Area Health Boards in Scotland and by the Central Services Agency on behalf of Health and Social Services Boards in Northern Ireland, give women's names, addresses and dates of births, as well as the names and addresses of their general practitioners. Although these registers are known to have a number of inaccuracies (up to 20 per cent of addresses may be inaccurate) they are the only source of the information required.

Invitations to be screened

7.4 Systems for inviting women to be screened for cervical cancer have already been developed, and can be adapted and enhanced for a breast cancer screening programme. In England and Wales the FPC will send to each general practitioner, at regular intervals, a list of those eligible for screening. The general practitioner will delete the names of any women for whom screening is contraindicated (eg because of illness), and return the list to the FPC. A computerised invitation letter will be sent, normally under the name of the general practitioner. The form of it will be for local decision. A reminder letter may be required for women who do not respond.

Non-invited women

7.5 Some women outside the invited age-group for screening will wish to be screened. Women aged 65 and over shoud be allowed to attend for screening but need not be recalled routinely. As the evidence that women younger than 50 benefit from screening is uncertain, we suggest that they should consult their general practitioner who, if he or she considers them at increased risk, may consult with the screening service (see Chapter 5).

Basic screening stage

7.6 Taking mammograms. Clinical responsibility for individual women being screened will be taken by a doctor experienced in the clinical aspects of breast cancer screening, who may be a consultant radiologist. The doctor will not need to be present at screening clinics. At every screening attendance each woman will complete a short questionnaire. Essential information includes date of birth, presence in either breast of a lump or distortion, and past surgery with position of scars recorded. These data will be entered into a computerised record system. Mammography will be performed by a specially trained radiographer. Following mammography the woman will be told how she can obtain the result of her test. Immediate processing of the films and assessment of their adequacy by experienced radiographers is unnecessary and reduces the throughput of women. Films may be transported to a central processing unit.

7.7 Reading mammograms. The purpose of basic screening is not to make a diagnosis but to separate the women into those who need further investigation and those who do not. Reading the basic screening mammograms must be the responsibility of the consultant radiologist, although the task can be devolved. Where film reading is devolved to non-radiologists they will be trained to refer all films that are not obviously negative to the radiologist. The radiologist will then decide how to classify the difficult or suspicious films. Films should be read separately from the clinic session, since pressure to give an opinion before a woman leaves the clinic has been shown to lead to a high recall rate, low specificity and sensitivity, and slowing of the throughput of women. The task of reading mammograms is greatly facilitated by use of a roller viewer with prior loading of films by a radiographic or clerical assistant.

7.8 Reading of mammograms will separate women into 3 groups: those with negative findings; those with positive findings requiring assessment; and those with inadequate films for making a decision. The first group will be eligible for routine recall after the appropriate interval; the second need assessment; and the third group will need to be recalled to the basic screening unit for further mammograms eg to clarify composite shadows. These are essentially part of the basic screen and should be performed in the basic screening unit rather than by the assessment team.

7.9 Notification of results. The doctor with clinical responsibility for screening women will also be responsible for notifying both the woman and her general practitioner of the result. Various methods can be used, however the arrangements must include a fail-safe mechanism to ensure follow-up of positive results (see paragraph 7.17).

7.10 Where a woman is found to have a mammographic abnormality or where she reports the presence of a breast lump or distortion, assessment is required. Depending on the prior wishes of the general practitioner the woman will be referred by the doctor responsible either to the general practitioner or directly to the specialist assessment team. In the latter case the general practitioner must be informed.

7.11 Location of basic screening unit. A basic screening unit may be static or mobile, and according to local circumstances may be sited either within a community health clinic or a hospital. Hospital-based units should be separate from the hospital diagnostic X-ray department because the organisation of a screening clinic requires a rapid throughput of well women with very different expectations from the patients undergoing diagnostic X-ray investigation. Films will not need to be processed and read where the women will be screened. There may be advantages in locating these functions within the hospital diagnostic X-ray department. Arrangements for transporting films from a basic screening unit to the processing and reading locations may be required. Mobile units will also require the support of a central base.

Assessment and biopsy

7.12 As indicated in paragraph 7.10 a woman requiring assessment may be referred to a specialist assessment team. The team may hold its clinic sessions either within a hospital or within the community health clinic (which may also contain a basic screening unit). Each clinic session will require the services of a clinician, a radiographer, a nurse and a receptionist, backed-up by a radiologist and a pathologist. A medical member of the team must be responsible for the following:

7.12.1 co-ordinating the results of these further investigations;

7.12.2 reaching a decision on the need for biopsy or treatment and making appropriate arrangements;

7.12.3 notifying the woman, general practitioner and the central screening office.

7.13 In Chapter 6 we concluded that, wherever possible, biopsies of impalpable lesions detected by a screening programme should be performed by a specialist team consisting of a surgeon, radiologist and pathologist with appropriate experience and skills. It is likely that the same radiologist and pathologist will also be part of the assessment team. The surgeon will be responsible for notifying the results of the biopsy to the patient's general practitioner and the central screening office.

7.14 Each basic screening unit will require a full-time administrative secretary supported by clerical staff both in the screening office and the FPC. Computer links between the screening office, the basic screening unit, FPC, and, possibly, the specialist assessment team will be needed. The administrative secretary will be responsible for scheduling appointments; maintenance of the record system, including filing of records and mammograms; and for correspondence, including notification of results and liaison between the various agencies involved. Provision of sufficient administrative and clerical staff is as vital to the efficiency of the screening programme as provision of staff for screening and assessment.

Screening records system

7.15 A screening record system should be developed to fulfill the following functions: (i) identification, invitation and recall of eligible women for screening; (ii) attendance for screening and results; (iii) monitoring the screening process; (iv) monitoring effectiveness. The system should be computerised with links to the appropriate population register.

7.16 **Identification, invitation and recall.** The FPC registers in England and Wales, and their equivalents in Scotland and Northern Ireland, form the basis for identification of eligible women, and, with computerisation, enable an invitation system to be implemented with the general practitioners' consent, both for initial screening and for subsequent routine repeat visits. It is expected that all these registers will be computerised by March 1988.

7.17 **Attendance for screening and results.** A basic simple record is required giving identification particulars, date of attendance, present breast symptoms and past breast surgery. This record will accompany the mammographic films to the film reader and the radiologist, who will be responsible for adding the screening opinion in terms of routine recall, repeat film or referral for assessment. The date of attendance and the result will be added to the woman's FPC record and will be used for scheduling her next attendance. Screening attendances and results from non-invited women should also be added to their FPC records. If the woman will be referred for assessment the record will be flagged to expect a final diagnosis and this will provide a check that the appropriate referral has taken place.

7.18 **Monitoring the screening process.** Linkage to local pathology registers and cancer registries is desirable so that the diagnosis of breast cancer can be added to the relevant woman's record, if this is not already known. Together with the records outlined above this will enable the following aspects of the process to be monitored: acceptance rates; self-referrals; cancers detected by screening; interval cancers; proportion of women referred for assessment; proportion biopsied; and incidence of breast cancer in non-accepters.

7.19 **Monitoring the effectiveness of screening.** This can be done approximately by examining trends in age-specific breast cancer mortality available from routine statistics. However, linkage of mortality data to screening data will enable a more precise and useful method of monitoring effectiveness, in that deaths from breast cancer can be categorized into those among women diagnosed by screening, those in interval cases, those in women who refused, and those in non-invited women. Linkage of both incidence and mortality data with screening records may be feasible if the NHS Central Register is computerised. Effectiveness should be monitored at both local and national levels.

Quality control of mammography

7.20 To achieve the high standards required in a mammographic screening service, meticulous quality control is mandatory. The consultant radiologist together with the medical physicist and radiographers, in accordance with normal practice, will be responsible for ensuring quality control in each basic screening unit. Consistent high quality results will require a quality assurance programme, which might be controlled by designating certain mammography departments as quality assurance reference centres. An outline of their functions is given in Annex F.

Radiation protection and monitoring

7.21 The radiation protection of both staff and those who will be screened will need to be secured and monitored in accordance with the Ionising Radiations Regulations (1985) and the Ionising Radiations (Protection of Persons Undergoing Medical Examination or Treatment) Regulations, presently in draft.

Management

7.22 The data presented in Chapter 8 suggest that basic screening units will serve populations generally larger than those of English district health authorities, or their equivalents in other UK countries, and that specialist assessment teams may serve an even larger catchment area. In areas including both urban and rural populations there may be advantages in co-ordinating the work of static and mobile units. It will be for health authorities to agree between themselves on local arrangements. It is, however, essential that every health authority or group of health authorities should designate one person with responsibility for the organisation, planning, and epidemiologcal monitoring of the breast cancer screening programme for a defined population of women. Ideally this person will be a specialist in community medicine, who will undertake this responsibility in addition to other duties in preventive medical care (eg cervical cancer screening) and health service planning. Alternatively the individual may have clinical responsibility within the programme.

7.23 The person designated will arrange the method of implementing screening; will deploy staff and ensure their adequate training; will set targets for intermediate assessment of the screening process such as acceptance rates, sensitivity, specificity and costs; will ensure that there is an appropriate record system to provide continuous routine monitoring of these factors; and will take appropriate action if the screening programme fails to meet these intermediate objectives.

7.24 Setting-up a breast cancer screening service will require substantial managerial effort. Considerable co-operation between health authorities or boards, hospital specialists, FPCs and general practitioners will be needed. There will be training needs to be met and there may be difficulties in attracting suitable staff to a relatively narrow field of practice. The specialist assessment teams will need careful organisation and co-operation between different authorities. Experience gained in the few existing breast cancer screening centres and the cervical cancer screening programme will be invaluable during the development of this new service.

Conclusions

7.25 While no one organisational solution for a screening programme is necessarily right for each health authority, a plan for a screening programme should include the following:

7.25.1 women in the target group should be sent a personal invitation from their general practitioner;

7.25.2 arrangements for recording results at the basic screen must include a fail-safe mechanism, to ensure that action is taken on all positive results;

7.25.3 every basic screening unit should have access to a specialist team for the assessment of screen-detected abnormalities;

7.25.4 a screening record system should be developed to identify, invite and recall women eligible for screening; to record attendance for screening and results; and to monitor the screening process and its effectiveness;

7.25.5 there should be adequate arrangements for quality control both within and between centres so that an acceptable standard of mammography can be maintained;

7.25.6 a designated person should be responsible for managing each local screening service. The person chosen would have managerial ability and is likely to have experience in community or preventive health care, although the radiological aspects must be the responsibility of a consultant radiologist. Setting-up a breast cancer screening service will require substantial managerial effort.

7.26 We can see considerable advantage in forming central bodies to advise Health Departments on the introduction of breast cancer screening programmes, to monitor their effectiveness and efficiency and to keep their progress under review. Such bodies might also advise their Health Departments on future policy.

8 Service requirements

Throughput of women screened

8.1 The manpower and equipment required depends on the number of women seen at each stage in the screening procedure, which in turn depends on screening policies and practice and on acceptance and referral rates.

8.2 Figure 8.1 illustrates the annual throughput of women throughout the UK in the initial 3 years of a screening programme with the following assumptions:

8.2.1 all women aged 50 to 64 are called for mammographic screening over the 3-year period;

8.2.2 70 per cent of these women attend;

8.2.3 10 per cent of attendances at basic screening units are by non-invited women;

8.2.4 another 10 per cent of attendances are by women recalled for further mammograms where the initial film was unsatisfactory or the findings equivocal;

8.2.5 referral rates are 10 per cent for assessment and 1.5 per cent for biopsy.

8.3 Figure 8.2 illustrates the annual throughput of women throughout the UK in the fourth and subsequent years when a screening programme has been established. It is based on the assumption that women are recalled for screening every 3 years. In these screening rounds, covering a 15-year age-band, 3/15 (20 per cent) of screens will be initial prevalent screens and 12/15 (80 per cent) will be repeat screens. It is assumed that 10 per cent of prevalent screens and 5 per cent of repeat screens will be referred for assessment, and that 1.5 per cent of prevalent screens and 1 per cent of repeat screens will require biopsy. In Edinburgh and Guildford only 0.5 per cent of repeat screens require biopsy but to allow for a 3-year as opposed to a 1-year interval we have given a larger estimate.

8.4 Varying the frequency of screening and/or age-groups screened would have a significant effect on the number of screening attendances. This is illustrated in Annex J, Figure J.1.

8.5 In 1,000 women of the target age-group 4.9 breast cancers are expected to arise in a 3-year period. The cancer detection rate at repeat screens has been estimated on the assumption that screening will detect 75 per cent of these ie 3.7 per 1,000 women. (In the Two Counties (Sweden) study screening detected 74 per cent of breast cancers expected to arise over a 30 month period).

8.6 Figures 8.3 and 8.4 illustrate in the same way the throughput of women at each stage in the screening procedure for the population covered by a basic screening unit in the initial prevalence period and in the fourth and subsequent years. There is a considerable range of uncertainty around the assumptions on which these figures are based, particularly on acceptance rates and on the basic screening unit's capacity. Annex H presents a sensitivity analysis, varying those assumptions around the estimates used in this chapter.

Figure 8.1   Estimated annual number of women in the UK undergoing different
              stages of the screening process in the initial 3 years of a programme

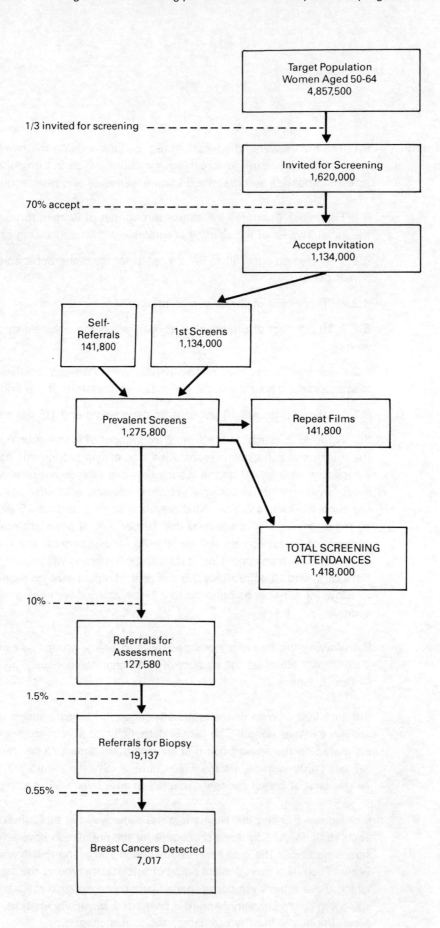

Figure 8.2   Estimated annual number of women in the UK undergoing different
             stages of the screening process in an established programme with
             a 3-yearly repeat screening cycle (4th and subsequent years).

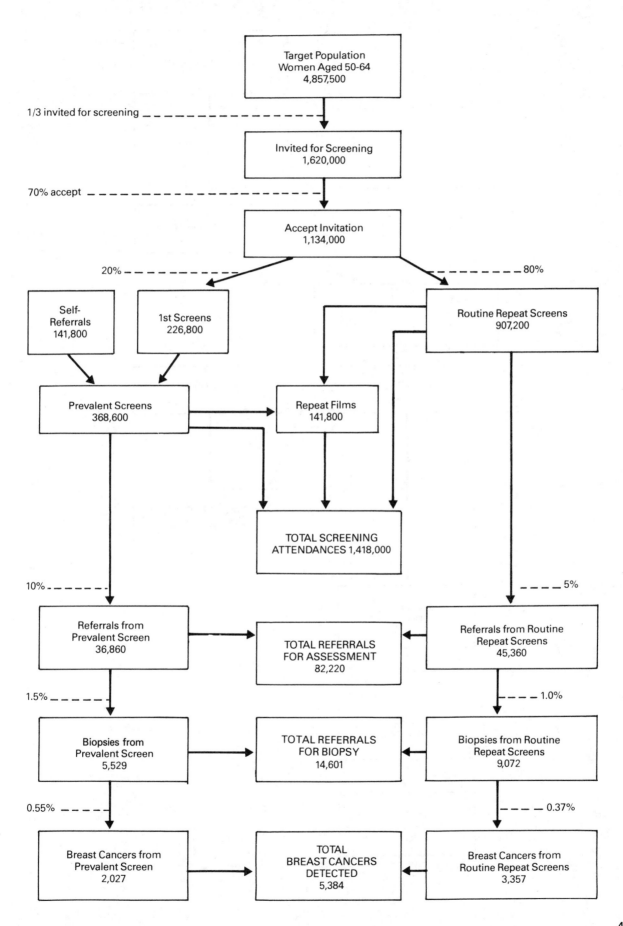

Figure 8.3

Estimated annual number of women undergoing different stages of the screening process in the initial 3 years of a programme in a population of 471,000 served by 1 basic screening unit.

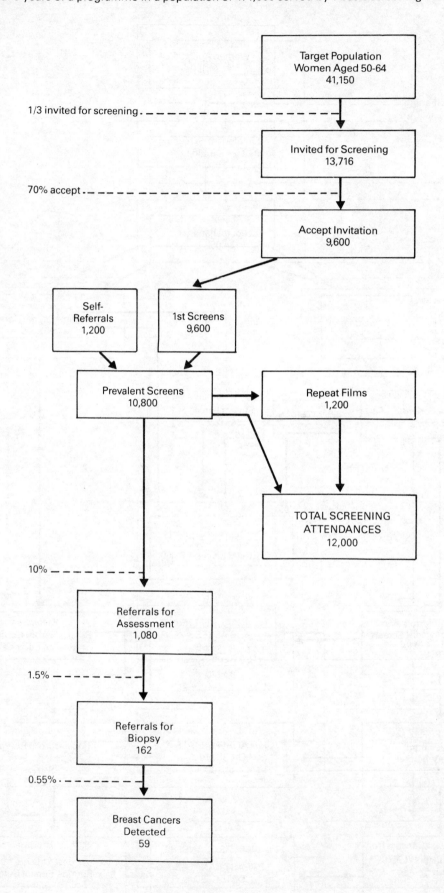

Figure 8.4   Estimated annual number of women undergoing different stages of the screening process in an established programme in a population of 471,000 served by 1 basic screening unit (4th and subsequent years).

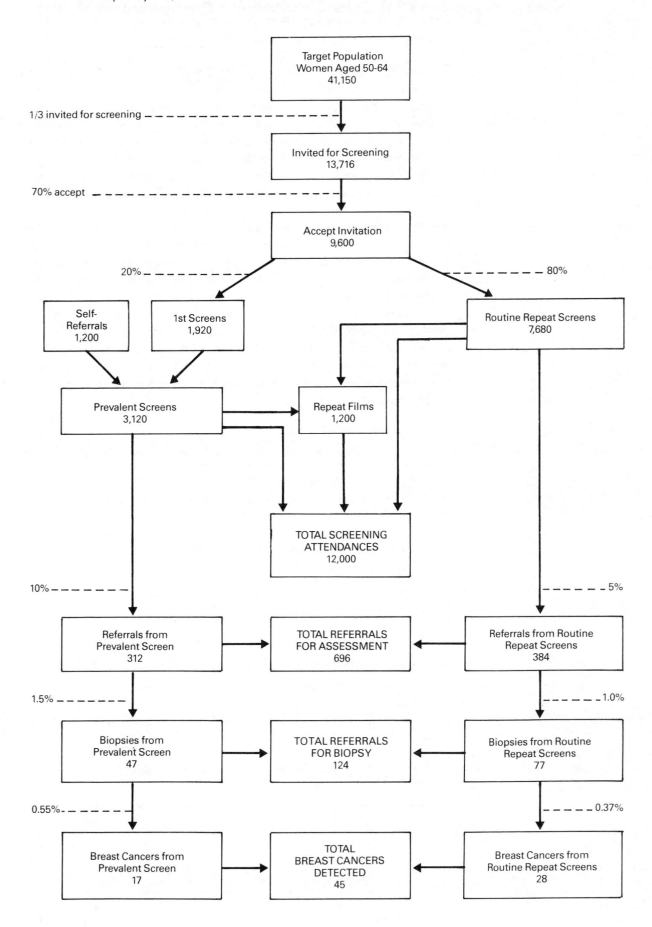

8.7 It is possible for a full-time screening unit with two radiographers and one mammography machine to take single-view mammograms of 40 women in each $3\frac{1}{2}$ hour session. This is reduced to 30 women if one radiographer works alone, and further reduced if two views are taken. In estimating service requirements we assume an average throughput of 30 women a session.

8.8 This could represent 300 women a week and 15,000 a year. Allowing for factors such as occasional equipment failure, unplanned staff absences and variations in the proportion of women who keep appointments, for example because of adverse weather, a realistic estimate of the annual throughput of each basic screening unit may be 12,000 women. Allowing for 10 per cent of total attendances to be by non-invited women and 10 per cent by women recalled for further views, each unit can cover a population of 41,150 women aged 50 – 64 within a total population of nearly half a million.

8.9 To estimate the extra workload generated by screening we need to know the workload in the absence of screening. We do not know the number of women in the target age-group who currently attend their general practitioners with breast symptoms, nor do we know the number of these women who are referred for further investigation. However, the number of biopsies in excess of those that would be necessary in the absence of screening can be estimated. The present number of biopsies in women in this age group is about 3.5 per 1,000 per annum. Table 8.1 (below) shows that in the first 3 years of a screening programme between 2 and 3 extra biopsies will be generated each week by each basic screening unit and that in the subsequent years only one extra biopsy will be generated each week.

Table 8.1 Estimated annual breast biopsy workload generated by a basic screening unit

A	Population of women aged 50 – 64 served by 1 basic screening unit	41,150
B	Expected number of breast biopsies in the absence of screening at a biopsy rate of 3.5 per 1,000	144
C	Expected number of breast biopsies during the first round of screening *Screened women at a biopsy rate of 15 per 1,000*	162
	Unscreened women (non-invited women and non-attenders) at a biopsy rate of 3.5 per 1,000	+111 =273
D	Expected number of breast biopsies during subsequent rounds of screening. *Screened women at a biopsy rate of 10–15 per 1,000*	124
	Women attending between screens at a biopsy rate of 1.75 per 1,000	+34
	Non-attenders at a biopsy rate of 3.5 per 1,000	+43 =201
E	Excess number of breast biopsies per annum during first screening round (C–B)	273 −144 =129
F	Excess number of breast biopsies per annum during subsequent screening rounds (D–B)	201 −144 = 57

Manpower implications

8.10 Each of the first three stages of the screening procedure (basic screening, assessment and biopsy) has implications for the numbers and training of staff employed from a number of professions. The manpower implications for radiologists and radiographers are critical to the introduction of a screening programme. It is essential that no centre should undertake screening without having a high level of expertise in mammography in order to minimise false-negative and false-positive findings. The training of staff and the maintenance of quality are important in all relevant disciplines and for all stages in the screening procedure. The requisite expertise will need to be spread progressively from existing centres.

8.11 **Existing expertise.** There are at present four levels of mammographic expertise in the UK.

8.11.1 Edinburgh and Guildford have been involved in population screening within the UK Trials for some years. We understand that in addition there are about 8 departments of radiology in the UK with skills in mammographic screening. Some are associated with active breast groups with facilities for assessment and biopsy.

8.11.2 In some further 15 departments mammography has been developed in association with active breast groups concerned with the management of symptomatic breast disease. The associated facilities required in the assessment and biopsy stages are likely to be well established in Districts or Boards containing these departments.

8.11.3 There are about 100 other departments that undertake some mammography although many of their machines are obsolete. Their staff will need considerable training and expansion to become sufficiently skilled to achieve the high quality of mammography necessary for screening and assessment. The availability and level of associated facilities is believed to be variable and would require correspondingly greater improvement than in the more experienced centres.

8.11.4 There are about 100 Districts or Boards that have no mammographic facilities.

8.12 **Assessment of manpower requirements.** In paragraph 8.8 we estimated that each basic screening unit could serve a population of 41,150 women aged 50–64 within a total population of nearly half a million. This implies a requirement of around 120 basic screening units throughout the UK. (The sensitivity of this estimate to different assumptions is analysed in Annex H). This is fewer than the number of Districts and Boards in the UK (219). In view of the shortage of trained staff and the cost of equipment, it would be more cost effective, if practicable, for each basic screening unit to serve the maximum population rather than to have one for each District or Board. We have estimated service requirements on this basis. The long-term manpower implications of screening the women served by a typical basic screening unit, and the total manpower implications for the UK based on 120 such units, are set out in Table 8.2.

8.13 The requirements described in paragraphs 8.14–8.23 reflect the experience of the Edinburgh and Guildford screening centres and give only a broad indication of the manpower likely to be required for a nation-wide service. The manpower pattern will vary across the country. Individuals with multidisciplinary skills may combine functions, for example clinical examination with film reading. Surgeons, radiologists, pathologists and radiographers will probably have other health service duties and may spend only a proportion of their time in a screening role.

Table 8.2 Summary of long-term manpower implications

						For all UK (120 basic screening units)
	For workload generated by each basic screening unit					
	Screening office /FPC	Basic screening unit	Assess-ment team	Additional biopsy workload	Total	Total
Radiologist		0.20*	0.15	0.05	0.40	48
Radiographer		1.50	0.15	0.05	1.70	204
Radiographic assistant		0.50			0.50	60
Clinician			0.15		0.15	18
Pathologist			0.05	0.05	0.10	12
Surgeon				0.05	0.05	6
Nurse			0.15	0.05	0.20	24
Receptionist/ Secretary		1.00	0.15		1.15	138
Administration) Clerical)	3.00				3.00	360
Driver		0.50			0.50	60
Total	3.00	3.70	0.80	0.25	7.75	930

* Alternatively, 0.10 for review only, if initial film reading is by a non-radiologist. The number of radiographers or clinicians would then need to be increased by 0.30 for film reading.

8.14 **Management.** We should expect that the individuals designated by each health authority or group of health authorities to be responsible for overall management of a local screening programme would normally have other responsibilities either in preventive medicine or within the screening procedure. However, these managers will require appropriate additional administrative and clerical support in a central screening office.

8.15 **Call and recall.** The operation of computerised call and recall systems based on population registers will require additional clerical support for despatch of invitations and updating of records. This support can be located either with the registers, for example at Family Practitioner Committees in England, or at the central screening office. Call and recall should not have manpower implications for general practices. Similarly, although general practitioners will probably be involved in post-screen counselling for some women, this should have no manpower implications.

8.16 A very broad estimate of the total administrative and clerical support at screening offices and for FPCs is 3 Whole Time Equivalents (WTE) per basic screening unit.

8.17 **Basic screening.** The minimum staff required to undertake one clinic session at a basic screening unit is one receptionist and one radiographer. Some further support from another radiographer, or possibly a radiographic assistant, is recommended: in Table 8.2 we allow for the Whole Time Equivalent of 1.5 radiographers. Local arrangements for other support can be made as necessary, eg to drive mobile units, to transport films to the film-reading location, and for periodic inspection of mammography machines by a medical physicist.

8.18 Assuming that a radiologist reads 110 films (55 women) an hour, a conservative allowance for film-reading is two consultant radiologist sessions a week, ie 0.2 WTE radiologists. Film-reading by non-radiologists at a rate of 80 films (40 women) an hour requires up to 3 sessions a week, plus up to one session by a radiologist to review mammograms that are not obviously normal. Processing films and loading them on to roller viewers prior to reading requires up to 5 radiographic assistant sessions a week.

8.19 **Assessment.** In Figure 8.4 we estimated that each basic screening unit would refer about 700 women to the specialist assessment teams a year or about 15 a week. If such teams were to work full-time seeing 10 women per session, and if every screening referral went to them, only 15−20 assessment teams would be required in the whole country. However, this would be impracticable both from the point of view of accessibility for the patients and of other commitments of the staff, particularly their hospital sessions. We anticipate that assessment teams will be developed in those centres with the necessary expertise, each working a sufficient number of sessions to provide for referrals from 1−3 basic screening units.

8.20 The staff to provide the services required for an assessment session is one clinician, one radiologist, one radiographer, one nurse and one receptionist/ secretary, plus about one hour from a pathologist.

8.21 Assuming that 10 women can be assessed in one session and that each basic screening unit refers an average of 15 women for assessment a week, each basic screening unit will generate three assessment sessions a fortnight, ie 0.15 WTE for each member of the team plus about 0.05 WTE pathologists.

8.22 **Biopsy.** Screening will lead to some increase in the number of biopsies, particularly during the prevalence round (although that would be spread over 3 years). In Table 8.1 we estimated that the additional biopsies generated by each basic screening unit would be some 57 a year in the long-term, and 129 in each of the first 3 years. This will increase workload not only because of the additional numbers but also because of the increased proportion of impalpable lesions requiring localisation. In practice we expect that workload will increasingly be concentrated on a relatively small number of surgeons and supporting teams, so that any overall increase will not be evenly distributed; this may present difficulties. In Table 8.2 we have included a long-term increase equivalent to 6 WTE for all of the UK for each of surgeons, radiologists, radiographers, pathologists and nurses.

8.23 **Treatment.** Screening is not likely to lead to a significant long-term increase in the number of women treated (see paragraph 6.18). During the prevalence round there will be an increase in the numbers treated and therefore in the workload of the relevant specialists, particularly surgeons and radiotherapists. We have not attempted to quantify the manpower implications as this increase in workload will be short-term.

8.24 **Training.** The numbers of individuals requiring training may be at least double the totals of radiologists and radiographers required because it is unlikely that in the long-term the same individuals will provide all the sessions required in one unit.

8.25 Paragraph 8.10 suggested that expertise be progressively spread throughout the UK from existing centres. Notes on a teaching programme based on existing centres are at Annex G. This would have manpower implications for the teaching centres during the development phase, but the effect on long-term national manpower requirements would be modest.

Building and equipment implications

8.26 **Basic screening unit.** The basic screening unit may be either static or mobile. Static and mobile units may work in combination. The static unit may be sited in a hospital or in a clinic in the community. Because of the rapid throughput of women for screening and because these are well women and not patients it is preferable that the unit is separate from the main hospital X-ray department. In addition to a mammographic room, space is also required for waiting, reception and changing. The mammographic room will house the mammographic machine and should have a single viewing box. A processing unit will be required, but this can serve the needs of more than one basic screening unit. The room for film reading need not be within the screening clinic, and to make best use of the radiologist's time there is some advantage in locating it in a diagnostic X-ray department.

8.27 **Mobile unit.** Mobile units will travel from a central base to spend appropriate periods sited near local community facilities. Water and electricity must be available to suit the requirements of the mammographic machine and film processor (if included) and to meet the heating and washing requirements of patients and staff. The mobile unit may be self-propelled or a caravan trailer, for which an appropriate towing vehicle is required. There is also a need for adjacent reception facilities. Fully equipped caravan trailers are available commercially and cost, at 1986 prices, about £35,000.

8.28 **Basic mammography machine.** The machine for basic screening need not be sophisticated. It need not have magnification facilities but a stationary grid may be provided. It costs, at 1986 prices, about £25,000. Film cassettes that minimise radiation absorption and maximise image quality should be used.

8.29 **Film processor.** Film processing is an important part of the image production chain. A dedicated processor with a development cycle and chemistry matched to the chosen film is required. Manufacturers are now providing 'matched' sets of films, intensifying screens, processors and chemicals. Ideally the processor cycle duration and chemistry temperature should be variable to allow for modification when improved films become available. A processor costs, at 1986 prices, about £6,000.

8.30 **Film viewer.** We have estimated that the films of 55 women might be read in 1 hour (paragraph 8.18). Reading at this speed requires a dedicated multi-film roller viewer, ideally fitted with blinds to minimise ambient light. It costs, at 1986 prices, about £10,000.

8.31 **Other major equipment.** The screening record system described in Chapter 7 requires computer facilities. The FPC call and recall systems that are already being computerised for cervical screening could readily be adapted and enhanced.

8.32 **Assessment and biopsy requirements.** The assessment techniques may be carried out either in a hospital or in a clinic in the community (paragraph 6.14). The assessment can probably be done by the specialist assessment team when other clinics are not being held and so would not require purpose-built accommodation.

8.33 The mammography machine required for assessment is a more sophisticated machine than that for basic screening. It should be equipped for magnification techniques and have an integral fixed or moving grid facility. A simple stereotactic accessory should ideally be available for the localisation techniques required for fine needle aspiration and later for the biopsy of impalpable screen-detected abnormalities. A mammography machine of this type costs, at 1986 prices, about £60,000.

8.34 If the technique of ultrasonography is used a hand-held, real-time ultrasound scanner should be sufficient. It costs, at 1986 prices, about £25,000.

8.35 A dedicated X-ray machine for specimen radiology is required by any specialist team undertaking biopsies of impalpable lesions. It costs, at 1986 prices, about £3,000.

8.36 **Existing Facilities.** Table 8.3 (below) gives the results of a survey we carried out in 1985 to identify the number of mammographic machines in the UK installed or upgraded since 1975. The numbers are divided between those with their own generator and those sharing a generator with other X-ray equipment. The latter are now considered obsolete. In the 219 Districts or Boards in the UK there are, according to our survey, only 128 machines that have their own generator. Almost all of these are used for the diagnosis of symptomatic patients.

Table 8.3 Existing Mammographic Facilities in the UK

Country	Regional Health Authority/Special Health Authority	Number of Districts/Boards	Number of Machines Installed or Upgraded since 1975		
			With Own Generator	Sharing Generator	Total
England	Northern	16	5	2	7
	Yorkshire	17	11	1	12
	Trent	12	6	3	9
	East Anglian	8	5	1	6
	North West Thames	14	6	2	8
	North East Thames	16	7	5	12
	South East Thames	15	10	2	12
	South West Thames	13	6	5	11
	Wessex	10	5	3	8
	Oxford	8	8	3	11
	South Western	11	4	4	8
	West Midlands	22	12	6	18
	Mersey	10	8	2	10
	North Western	19	8	—	8
	Total	191	101	39	140
	The Royal Marsden Hospital		3	—	3
	Total	191	104	39	143
Scotland		15	11	8	19
Wales		9	7	7	14
Northern Ireland		4	6	1	7
Total		219	128	55	183

Source: Survey conducted by the DHSS for the Working Group in 1985.

8.37 **Capital investment requirements.** If the capital expenditure on equipment and buildings that has been identified in the Edinburgh economic study were replicated throughout the UK it would total some £31 million at 1985–86 prices (see Chapter 9). However, costs can be expected to vary depending on a number of factors including the extent to whch existing facilities can be used, and the balance between static and mobile units.

8.38 The 10 departments of radiology described in 8.11 as having screening expertise should require the least capital investment. However, the only mobile screening units identified from our survey are at the Edinburgh and Guildford UK trial centres. If mobile units are required more capital investment will be needed.

8.39 The 15 departments in which mammography has been developed would probably need to invest in building alterations and screening equipment. Their existing facilities could probably then be used for assessment.

8.40 The 100 departments that provide limited mammographic facilities would require much more capital investment.

8.41 It is likely that many of the Districts/Boards that have no existing facilities will arrange with neighbouring authorities to share their facilities for basic screening and assessment.

Conclusions

8.42 **The manpower implications for radiologists and radiographers are critical to the introduction of a screening programme. No centre should undertake screening without having a high level of expertise in mammography in order to minimise false-negative and false-positive findings.**

8.43 **The training of staff and the maintenance of quality is important in all relevant disciplines and for all stages in the screening procedure. The requisite expertise will need to be spread progressively from existing centres.**

8.44 **A basic screening unit, screening 12,000 women a year, could serve a population of some 41,500 women aged 50–64 within a total population of nearly half a million. This implies a requirement for around 120 basic units throughout the UK. This is fewer than the number of Districts and Boards in the UK (219). In view of the shortage of trained staff and the cost of equipment, it would be more cost effective, if practicable, for each basic screening unit to serve the maximum population rather than to have one for each District or Board.**

8.45 **Specialist assessment teams should be developed in those Districts or Boards with the necessary expertise in breast cancer diagnosis, each team working a sufficient number of sessions to provide for referrals from 1–3 basic screening units.**

8.46 **An established UK breast cancer screening programme with 120 basic screening units will require some 930 Whole Time Equivalent staff including about 40 radiologists and about 200 radiographers.**

8.47 **In practice, both biopsies and treatments will increasingly be concentrated on a relatively small number of surgeons and supporting assessment teams, so that any overall increase in workload will not be evenly distributed.**

8.48 Training of radiologists and radiographers will have some manpower implications in the development phase of a screening programme but these should be negligible in the long-term.

8.49 Introducing a screening programme will initially require substantial capital investment in equipment and buildings. A mobile unit may, in some circumstances, be the preferred option for basic screening.

9 Economic appraisal

Introduction

9.1 In this chapter we draw together the limited information on the costs and benefits of screening for breast cancer by mammography. The key concepts of economic appraisal are set out below. The main costs and benefits are categorised and described in paragraphs 9.14–9.23, with best estimates of the magnitudes of these costs and benefits. Thereafter, we focus attention on the overall implications of screening for NHS resources and for comparisons with other uses of health service resources.

Economic appraisal

9.2 Economic appraisal is a general term for a set of techniques which are used to compare the relative efficiency of alternative ways of using society's scarce resources. Three approaches can be used to answer different questions: cost-effectiveness analysis (CEA), cost-benefit analysis (CBA), and cost-utility analysis (CUA).

9.3 **Cost-Effectiveness Analysis (CEA).** CEA is employed when the problem is one of achieving a given objective at least cost or of maximising a given output from a fixed budget. That the objective is worthwhile is not open to question in this form of analysis. It is also limited to considering 'single output' policies. Applied to screening for breast cancer, CEA can address issues such as which screening method has the lowest cost per true positive detected. As such CEA is of limited use in appraising screening programmes.

9.4 **Cost-Benefit Analysis (CBA).** The purpose of CBA is to assist in answering questions concerning whether or not different activities are worthwhile. In order to do this, ideally all the costs and all the benefits have to be identified, measured and valued in commensurate (ie money) terms. If costs outweigh benefits then there are no economic grounds for pursuing the activity.

9.5 **Cost-Utility Analysis (CUA).** The inherent difficulties of valuing changes in mortality and morbidity in money terms have led to the development of a hybrid approach labelled as CUA. The objective is to make the outcomes of health projects commensurate with one another by measuring outcomes in terms of life-years gained, ideally adjusted for quality. All other costs and benefits are valued in money terms and projects can be ranked against each other in terms of net cost per life-year or quality-adjusted-life-year (QALY) gained. This approach can of course be applied to projects that enhance life rather than extend it. The limitation of CUA is that it cannot help, directly, to answer questions of how much should be spent on individual health care projects. However, it can be used to assist consideration of whether screening for breast cancer contributes more per £ spent to the improvement of health than other competing uses.

9.6 **Opportunity cost.** This latter point is clearly of importance in attempting to ensure that the maximum benefit is achieved from the resources available to the health service. It is for this reason that economists put great emphasis on the concept of opportunity cost; that is, the value of other opportunities which are forgone when resources are used in one particular way. Formally, the opportunity cost is defined as the value of the best alternative which is forgone. If the benefits of a project exceed the opportunity cost, then we can be confident that there is no other allocation of resources that will produce a greater benefit to society.

9.7 It is reasonable to assume that the opportunity cost of introducing breast cancer screening would be in terms of other health-related projects, whatever the size of the overall budget. The CUA approach enables comparisons to be made with some possible competing uses of resources, for which cost per life-year or cost per quality-adjusted-life-year calculations have been carried out.

9.8 **Marginal costs and benefits.** In order to determine the best scale of activity for any service, it is important to consider the marginal costs and benefits; that is, the costs and benefits that result from doing a little bit more of something or a little bit less. Although attention is focussed in this chapter on the broad aggregates involved in breast cancer screening, the costs and benefits will vary according to which women are screened, how often and by what method or combination of methods. Data to consider these issues will emerge from the economic evaluation being conducted in association with the UK trials. Some results on the marginal costs of combinations of screening methods are presented in Annex E.

9.9 **Discounting.** When costs and benefits occur in different time periods, as they will with screening, discounting becomes important. Costs and benefits that occur in the future are given less weight than costs or benefits that occur now. This can be thought of either in investment terms or in terms of time preference. Costs (or benefits) in the future are discounted because a smaller cash amount could be invested now and accumulate interest to meet the future cost (or to compensate for the future benefit). Discounting also gives expression to the fact that people may have a straight preference for benefits sooner rather than later (and costs later rather than sooner). A 5 per cent discount rate is employed here.

Our approach

9.10 The results presented here are based on a CUA approach to the evaluation of screening by mammography. They represent the best estimates presently available but should be treated cautiously. The information available to us on the costs and benefits of screening by mammography was necessarily limited to data from the overseas trials and the data starting to emerge from the UK trials. Economic studies linked to the UK trials are still in progress.

Studies reported

9.11 We have obtained most of the cost figures in this report from an economic study by health economists P R Clarke and N Fraser which has been costing the screening service provided in Edinburgh as part of the UK trial of breast cancer screening (see Selected Bibliography (8)). These figures have been supplemented by some preliminary information from the economic study that began in the English trial centres last year.

9.12 The UK trials are not due to report their findings on outcome until 1988. Therefore, all data on the outcome of screening have been taken from the published results of trials carried out elsewhere. Data from the Two Counties (Sweden) study have been used for measuring outcomes in the first 9 years after the screening programme commenced, because this study is the most recent. The longer-term effect of screening has been extrapolated from the HIP (New York) study and is, necessarily, based on a much older study.

9.13 Two of the European studies, Two Counties (Sweden) and Nijmegen (Netherlands), have reported on the economic implications of screening. However, the differences in health service costs between these countries and the UK are such that the results are unlikely to be of any direct relevance. (See Selected Bibliography (18)(48)).

Identifying the costs and benefits

9.14 The costs and benefits of screening can usefully be considered in relation to four groups of women screened: women with no disease and a negative screen (true negatives); women with asymptomatic disease and a positive screen (true positives); women with asymptomatic disease and a negative screen (false negatives); and women with no disease and a positive screen (false positives). A final group consists of those women who do not attend. A brief outline of the costs and benefits for each group is given in Table 9.1 (below).

Table 9.1 Costs and benefits by screening category (excluding psychological factors)

Screening Category	Costs	Benefits
a. True negatives	Cost of screening.	
b. True positives	Cost of screening.	QALYs gained compared with not screening
	* Cost of any additional cases treated as a result of screening.	* Possible saving on treatment cost due to earlier stage at treatment.
	* Cost of treating cases earlier (effect of discounting) and cost of longer post-treatment follow up.	
c. False negatives	Cost of screening.	
	* Cost due to any subsequent delay in seeking treatment.	
d. False positives	Cost of screening.	
	Cost of assessment and biopsy.	
e. Non-attenders	Costs of invitation (if call and recall scheme operated).	

* These items have not been included in the subsequent analysis.

9.15 In estimating the costs and benefits, consideration should be given to those accruing to the NHS, to other public sector agencies, to the patient and family and to the rest of society.

Cost to the NHS

9.16 **The Basic Screen.** The main cost to the NHS is the provision of the basic screen since this is provided for a large number of women. The cost per woman screened by single view mammography (including assessment of suspicious results) has been estimated as £11.66 (see Annex E). All administrative costs (eg for call and recall) are included but current screening programmes notify women of positive results only. Notifying results to all women would increase the basic cost.

9.17 **Biopsy.** In the initial (prevalence) screening round there will be increased costs for investigation of *additional* women with abnormalities ie over and above those who would present in the absence of screening. Although the costs of individual procedures may be large, there will be relatively few cases in comparison with the number of women screened. The number of false positives who are investigated will depend upon the specificity of the basic screen and the ability of the assessment procedures to reduce the number requiring biopsy. With annual rescreening, costs for subsequent rounds have been almost identical to those for the control population. It is not known what the biopsy costs in subsequent rounds will be with a longer screening interval. In the analysis presented later it has been assumed that they are the same as for the prevalence screen, ie a biopsy rate for 3-yearly incidence screens of 1.5 per cent whereas in Chapter 8 we assumed 1 per cent.

9.18 **Treatment.** Although the initial (prevalence) screening round will result in additional numbers of women with breast cancer being treated, no attempt has been made to include any costing of this. The numbers involved will be small (about one case a week from each basic screening unit) and it seems likely that the increase in the surgical and radiotherapy workload would be modest, especially if the prevalence screen were to be spread over three years. Most of these women would have been treated sooner or later in the absence of screening. The only potential source of a general increase in cases for treatment would seem to be from cancers that would not otherwise present clinically; for example, because of death from another cause occurring prior to any symptoms arising. The chance of this happening will increase as the upper age for screening increases. The numbers are likely to be small so that there would be no significant effect on total costs. (In the HIP (New York) study there was no excess of cases at 7 years but latest figures from Sweden show an excess at 6 years.)

Costs to other public sector agencies

9.19 There are no data available on costs to other public sector agencies arising from screening but it seems unlikely that there would be any significant changes.

Cost to patients

9.20 **Time and travel.** Attendance for screening involves women in costs for travel to the clinic or screening venue. There is also a time cost, which may involve a loss of either work or leisure time. Some estimates of cost to women are given in Annex E. Time spent being screened will vary with the organisation of the clinic and the effort made to reduce waiting times. Travel costs will depend on local geography and may be reduced by initiatives such as mobile mammography units.

9.21 **Psychological factors.** The process of undergoing screening is likely to involve some additional adverse effects for women, particularly those in the false positive group, due to the anxiety which may be induced by screening. However, after the screening has taken place, there may be a reassurance value. Although it is possible, in theory, to estimate a value for such psychological factors, no work has yet been carried out on this issue. Indeed, there is no hard evidence to say whether there is a net cost or net benefit to be considered.

Benefits

9.22 **Reduced mortality.** Extending the life expectancy of the women with screen-detected cancer is the direct benefit from the screening programme. Until the UK trials report, the only available data on reduced mortality are those from the Two Counties (Sweden) trial (mammography only) and from the HIP (New

York) trial (mammography and clinical examination). Figure 9.1 (opposite) illustrates the results for the two trials mentioned (see Selected Bibliography (2)(33)(34)(37). It should be noted that in the HIP (New York) trial screening was discontinued after the trial period of four screening rounds.

9.23 **Production gains.** Apart from the intrinsic value of extending life, the gain in healthy years of life also benefits society through the contribution made to productive output during the years gained. It should be stressed that there may be a gain regardless of whether or not the person whose life is extended is in paid employment. Housework, for example, has a value even though it is not paid for.

Cost per life-year gained

9.24 In order to summarise the costs and benefits of breast cancer screening in a way that is readily comparable with other uses of health service resources, estimates have been made of the cost per life-year gained and the cost per QALY. While there are many possible types of screening and methods of organising screening this exercise is necessarily limited by the fact that suitable outcome data are currently available only from overseas trials, and comprehensive costing data are available only for one UK location, Edinburgh. Our suggested screening programme (Chapter 8) does not correspond exactly to any of the trials that have been carried out.

9.25 Given these limitations, the estimates presented here are nonetheless of the correct order of magnitude and therefore useful as indicators. Efforts have been made to indicate the kind of variation in these results that can be expected when different factors are taken into account. The estimates presented here are all based on NHS costs per life-year gained or QALY. Although other costs and the productive value of life years gained should ideally be included, most other studies of this kind have included only health service costs. Therefore, the estimates have been made as comparable as possible.

9.26 **The base estimate.** The base estimate for the cost per life-year gained has been calculated by taking cost estimates for our suggested screening programme with screening by single-view mammography only at 3-year intervals. Three screening rounds have been included; in the overseas trials, data from 3 screening rounds in Sweden have been published and 4 from the HIP (New York) study. The acceptance rate is assumed to be 70 per cent for the initial round and to fall by 1 per cent per annum for subsequent rounds. Life-years gained have been estimated by extrapolating the results of the Swedish trial from 9 years to 15 years, using the experience of the HIP (New York) study as the basis for this extrapolation. This base estimate produces a discounted cost per life-year gained of **£3,044.** (Details of this calculation are given in Annex K as an example of the process). A second estimate has been produced which includes an allowance for the cost of screening uninvited women. Under the extreme assumption that no extra benefit is generated, the discounted cost per life-year is **£3,391.**

9.27 **Changing the time horizon.** The decision about when to terminate the calculation of the life-years gained is not straightforward. The results of extrapolation are more unreliable the further they are taken but an early cut-off point may over-estimate the costs per life-year gained. Figure 9.2 shows how the cost per life-year gained varies with the estimate duration of the number of years of benefit, based on extrapolation of the Swedish results. The choice of 15 years for the base estimate does not seem too unreasonable, as the impact of extending the time horizon is tailing off after this point.

Figure 9.1   Mortality results from overseas trials

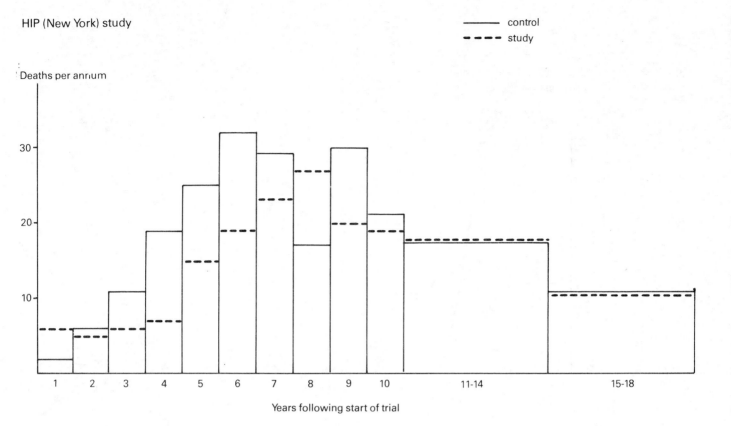

HIP (New York) study

——— control
- - - study

Deaths per annum

Years following start of trial

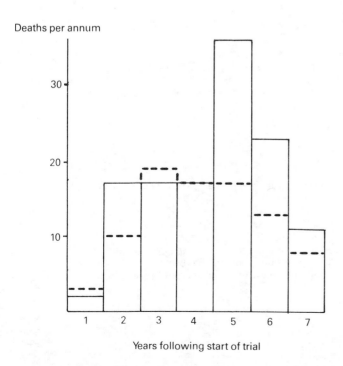

Two counties (Sweden) study

Deaths per annum

Years following start of trial

The histograms above show the annual number of deaths from breast cancer in the HIP (New York) study and the Two Counties (Sweden) study. No woman had had breast cancer diagnosed on entry to the studies. Despite the different design of the two studies the histograms show that by year 5 both had achieved a mortality reduction.

Figure 9.2   Variation of cost per life-year gained with the estimated years of benefit.

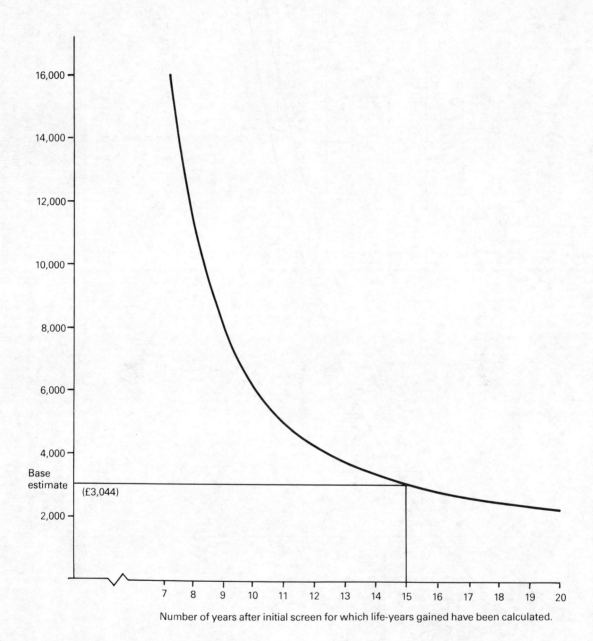

The cost per life-year gained for women found to have breast cancer by mammographic screening depends on the number of years for which the benefit is considered to last. This graph has been constructed by extrapolating the data from the Two Counties (Sweden) study, and shows that if the benefit lasts for 15 years the discounted cost per life-year gained is £3,044.

Figure 9.3   Variation of cost per life-year gained with the effectiveness of a screening programme.

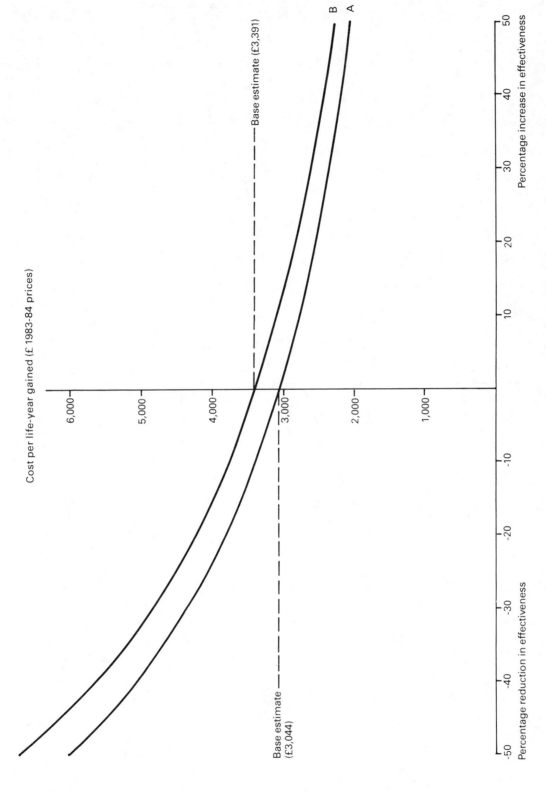

Assuming that the benefit of detecting breast cancer by mammographic screening tests lasts for 15 years, the above graph shows how the cost per life-year gained for a target population of women aged 50-64, would vary if the programme was either more or less effective in prolonging life than was the Two Counties (Sweden) study (line A). The graph also shows (line B) the impact of taking into account the cost of screening women who have not been invited with the extreme assumption of no extra benefit being generated.

Figure 9.4   Variation of cost per quality-adjusted-life-year gained (QALY) with the effectiveness of a screening programme.

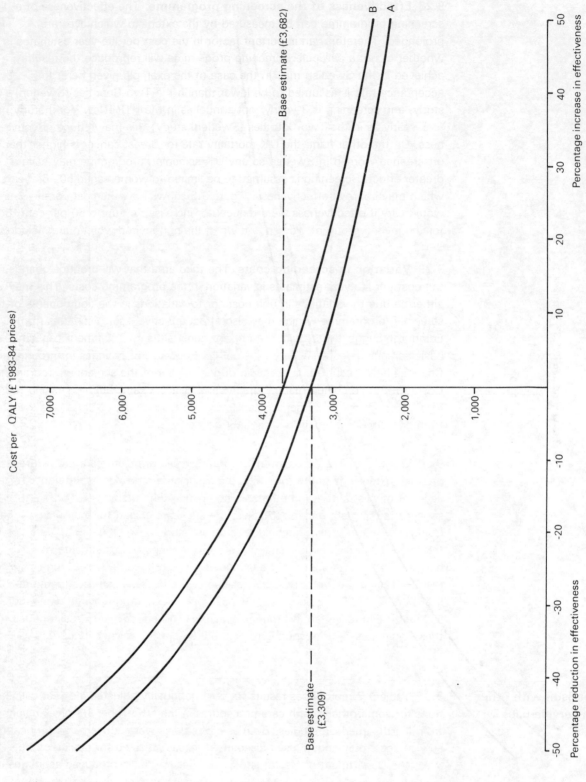

Cost per   QALY (£ 1983-84 prices)

The above graph is a variation on Figure 9.3 incorporating a correction factor that takes into account the morbidity that may accompany the natural history and the treatment of breast cancer. The resulting measure is the cost per quality-adjusted-life-year gained (QALY). Line A refers to the target screening population, while line B includes non-invited women with the extreme assumption of no extra benefit being generated

9.28 **Effectiveness of the screening programme.** The effectiveness of a screening programme can be measured by the extent to which lives are prolonged. Therefore, an important factor in the cost per life-year estimates is whether or not a particular screening programme will reproduce the results achieved in the Swedish trial. In the case of the example given here, the acceptance rate is assumed to be lower than in the Two Counties (Sweden) study, and screening is 3-yearly, not annual as in the HIP (New York) study or 2 to 3-yearly as in the Two Counties (Sweden) study; this may reduce effectiveness. On the other hand the UK mortality rate for breast cancer is higher than in unscreened women in Sweden so any UK screening programme may have a greater effect. Screening is assumed to be limited to women aged 50–64 years which may improve effectiveness. Figure 9.3 shows how the cost per life-year would vary if effectiveness were reduced or increased by up to 50 per cent, both for the invited group of women and when the non-invited women are included.

9.29 **Variation in screening costs.** The third area that will produce changes in the cost per life-year estimates is variation in the programme costs. This may either be due to variations in unit costs or to variations in the components of the screening programme (which may also affect effectiveness). Estimates from Edinburgh suggest that, with the present constraints on equipment capacity, basic screening cost may vary by 4 per cent because of changes in throughput. Changes have occurred, in practice, during the life of the screening programme. Costs for the combined mammography and clinical examination screening round have fallen from £16.23 per woman to £12.86 per woman because of a switch from two view to single view mammography.

9.30 **Quality of life adjustment.** Different types of health care procedures may produce extensions of life for which the associated morbidity is different. To take account of this factor, and others, in comparing the outcomes for different services, attempts are made to adjust the life-years gained for the quality of life. Using the Rosser scaling technique, a recent study on the quality of life following treatment for breast cancer suggested that the range of adjustments was between 0.92 and 0.99; other techniques have produced a wider range of results. Taking the worst possible case as 0.92, the base estimate (paragraph 9.26) becomes **£3,309** per QALY (**£3,682** per QALY if non-invited women are included). Figure 9.4 shows the impact of varying effectiveness assumptions for these estimates; it corresponds to Figure 9.3 adjusted for quality of life.

Comparison with other health service uses

9.31 Table 9.2 reproduces results for cost per quality-adjusted life-year calculations for some other health care procedures in the UK. Table 9.3 gives results from North American studies. Both sets of studies were concerned with health service costs only and all used discounted results adjusted for quality of life. Also, the Department of Health and Social Security have produced estimates of cost per life-year gained for screening for cervical cancer: the central estimate from a range of results is **£3,750** per life year (the range reflects uncertainty about the epidemiology of the disease). It can be seen, from the studies on dialysis for example, that costs in North America will generally be higher than in the UK and this should be taken into account when interpreting the results. While the estimates for cost per life-year or cost per QALY gained for breast cancer screening are not dissimilar to other health service activities currently undertaken, it is possible that expansion of certain other services may offer higher returns on resources spent. It should be noted that these results are based on the costs of present levels of activity and the marginal cost of increasing activities beyond certain levels may be higher (and the marginal benefit lower).

Table 9.2 Comparison of costs per Quality-Adjusted-Life-Year (QALY) gained for various health care procedures

Procedure	Value of the extra costs per QALY (£1983/84 prices)
Pacemaker implantation for atrioventricular heart block	700
Hip replacement	750
Coronary artery bypass grafting (CABG) for main vessel disease	1,040
Kidney transplantation	3,000
	Breast cancer screening estimated by working group to fall in this range
Heart transplantation	5,000
CABG for moderate angina with one vessel disease	12,000
Hospital haemodialysis	14,000

Source: Williams, A. (1985). Economics of coronary artery bypass grafting. British Medical Journal 291, 326–329.

Table 9.3 Comparative cost-utility results for selected programmes[a]

Programme	Reported cost/QALY[b] gained in US dollars (year)	Adjusted[c] cost/QALY[b] gained in US dollars 1983
PKU screening (phenylketonuria)	<0 (1970)	<0
Post-partum anti-D (rhesus incompatibility)	<0 (1977)	<0
Ante-partum anti-D (rhesus incompatibility)	1,220 (1983)	1,220
Coronary artery bypass surgery for left main coronary artery disease	3,500 (1981)	4,200
Neonatal intensive care, 1000–1499g	2,800 (1978)	4,500 Breast cancer screening estimated by working group to fall in this range
T4 (thyroid) screening	3,600 (1977)	6,300
Treatment of severe hypertension (diastolic ≧ 105mm Hg) in males age 40	4,850 (1976)	9,400
Treatment of mild hypertension (diastolic 95–104mm Hg) in males age 40	9,880 (1976)	19,100
Estrogen therapy for postmenopausal symptoms in women without a prior hysterectomy	18,160 (1979)	27,000
Neonatal intensive care, 500–999g	19,600 (1978)	31,800
Coronary artery bypass surgery for single vessel disease with moderately severe angina	30,000 (1981)	36,300
School tuberculin testing programme	13,000 (1968)	43,700
Continous ambulatory peritoneal dialysis	35,100	47,100
Hospital haemodialysis	40,200 (1980)	54,000

a. These studies use similar, but not identical, methods. Generally costs are net health care costs; however, discount rates and preference weights are not completely consistent. Differences in methods should be considered when comparing the relative cost-utility. Table taken from Torrance and Zipursky (1984).

b. QALY denotes Quality-Adjusted-Life-Year.

c. Adjusted to 1983 dollars according to the US Consumer Price Index for Medical Care for all urban consumers. Source: US Bureau of Labor Statistics, Monthly Labor Review.

Source: GW Torrance (1986). Measurement of health state utilities for economic appraisal. Journal of Health Economics 5, 1–30.

Table 9.4 Estimated revenue and capital costs of screening

	1983–84 prices			1985–86 prices	
	Basic Screening Unit	UK Total		UK Total	
	Based on central assumption	Based on central assumptions	Range	Based on central assumptions	Range
	£	£ million	£ million	£ million	£ million
Revenue Cost	135,000	16	13–20	18	15–22
Capital Cost					
— Equipment	115,000	14	10–18	15	11–20
— Buildings	120,000	14	11–19	16	12–21

Notes

1. Costs of basic screening unit includes costs of assessment and additional biopsies.

2. The range of costs are based on different assumptions for throughput and acceptance rates (see Annex H).

Implications for the NHS

9.32 Table 9.4 summarises the likely costs to the NHS of introducing the breast cancer screening programme described in Chapters 5, 7 and 8 (including costs of additional biopsies). These estimates for aggregate cost are in broad terms, of course, and it is unlikely that the unit costs derived for this report would be exactly replicated elsewhere. In particular, the overheads for running a screening service would be largely fixed regardless of the throughput, within the range considered here. Annex H presents some estimates of how the costs might vary under different assumptions about throughput and about acceptance rates.

9.33 Apart from the overheads element, there are other factors that may affect these cost estimates. In particular, assumptions have been made about the life of buildings and equipment that may not be realised in practice. Equipment costs have been discounted over 7 years and building costs over 30 years. Any variation in these assumptions would have an effect on costs. Also, it should be recognised that whilst any use of buildings is likely to have an opportunity cost there may not be any financial outlay if existing space can be used. Finally, the cost of biopsies will depend on the mix of techniques used; in particular, the number of biopsies done under general rather than local anaesthetic.

9.34 Table 9.4 separates out the revenue and capital elements of the cost estimates. Based on the experience at Edinburgh, the revenue costs for a single basic screening unit would be around £135,000, equipment costs might be up to £115,000 (with replacement possibly every 5–10 years), and the element allowed for buildings was £120,000 (with replacement possibly every 30 years). The gross equivalents for the UK are also shown in Table 9.4. The sensitivity analysis in Annex H suggests that the possible range around these estimates may be quite wide depending upon the assumptions used. The financial outlay for buildings will, of course, be less if existing space can be utilised. Also, the equipment costs for Edinburgh may not be typical of those for a basic screening unit. Some costs may have been incurred in setting up the study (pathology equipment, for example) which may not have to be met elsewhere. Actual equipment costs are likely to be very dependent on local circumstances and it should be possible for lower equipment costs to be achieved. There may be some substitution between the equipment and buildings costs if some areas introduced a mobile screening service.

Implications of extending the service

9.35 The cost estimates presented have taken account of up to 10 per cent women attending for screening who were not invited. The screening service could possibly absorb some additional workload at marginal cost (£3.56 per screen for single view mammography plus any assessment or biopsy costs). However, more frequent screening (eg biennial) or extending the service to a much wider age range, would require an increase in the number of basic screening units and, therefore, costs would increase pro rata. Thus, the cost for biennial screening would be approximately 50 per cent higher than the cost of screening every 3 years. An almost proportional increase in costs for major increases in the screening service seems to be a reasonable assumption but there are no data on the effect that this would have on benefits (life-years gained). Therefore, the cost per life-year gained for such changes cannot be calculated but it is hoped that such data can be obtained in the future.

Conclusions

9.36 The estimates for cost per life-year or cost per QALY gained for breast cancer screening are not dissimilar to other health service activities currently undertaken. It is possible that expansion of certain other services may offer higher returns on resources spent.

9.37 We estimate that the annual revenue cost to the NHS in the UK for running a screening service, based on the Edinburgh experience and with the parameters we suggest, is about £18 million (1985–86 prices). The capital cost is likely to be at most £31 million (1985–86 prices). More frequent screening or extending the service to a much wider range would require an increase in the number of basic units and, therefore, costs would increase *pro rata*.

10　Research

Introduction

10.1 Our conclusions on the effectiveness of screening for breast cancer rest upon the results of two large-scale overseas randomised trials and supporting population-based studies. Results from the UK Trial of Early Detection of Breast Cancer, which start to become available in 1988, will provide useful information on the effectiveness of breast cancer screening within a UK setting. In this chapter we discuss outstanding research needs which we believe must be addressed in parallel with the evolution of a screening service.

Screening intervals

10.2 Paramount in any programme of screening is the need to determine the optimum interval between episodes of screening. Following a prevalence screen some cases of undetected cancer will remain and new cases will develop. The optimum frequency of screening is therefore related to the sensitivity of the basic screen as well as the incidence rate of breast cancer. Good prospective studies are necessary to determine this interval.

Age

10.3 The optimum frequency of screening may not be the same for all women and the opportunity should be taken to explore relevant factors. The effect of varying intervals between screens in women of different age groups is one example.

10.4 There is no firm evidence that screening is effective for women under 50 years of age. Whilst a long-term objective is to find an effective method of screening these younger women, there is justification for further trials of existing methods of screening them. In view of the numbers this will require a multicentre study.

Risk factors

10.5 So far, studies of those factors that affect the risk of a woman developing breast cancer have not been successful in defining a high-risk population of women. Further epidemiological, radiological, biochemical and immunological work is clearly required.

10.6 At the same time primary prevention must be regarded as an ideal long-term aim, and, should it be possible to identify a subgroup of women at high risk, the mounting of interventional studies should be considered.

Improving acceptance

10.7 There is a need to identify those factors that influence a woman's response to an invitation to be screened and possible causes of anxiety generated by a screening programme. Similarly, the reasons why women continue to present to their doctors with long-standing and advanced disease require further study.

Screening methods

10.8 Little is known about the effectiveness of clinical examination or breast self-examination (BSE) as sole methods of basic screening. The UK trial will provide evidence of the effectiveness of BSE and of using clinical examination and mammography combined. It is important that the follow-up to the trial should continue until definitive results are obtained. In women over 50 years of age it is most unlikely that new studies involving a non-screened control group will be set up. Although it will therefore not be feasible to examine the effectiveness of clinical examination alone in this age group, it will be feasible to conduct studies in which the marginal costs and benefits of adding BSE or clinical examination to mammography can be determined. It will also be important to determine the role of BSE in the early detection of interval cancers. This is particularly important in view of the proposed initial frequency of screening of three years.

10.9 Currently mammography is the most effective method for the detection of early breast cancer. There is no study that compares the costs and benefits of single versus two-view mammography as a basic screening method. It is of interest that in Sweden, where single-view mammography has been successfully applied, two-views are recommended for the prevalence screen in their proposed national programme.

10.10 If mammography is to remain the standard method of early detection, further work will be needed on computer processing, storage and recall of mammographic images. At the same time work should proceed on alternative methods of imaging, eg ultrasonography and microwave thermography. Because of non-homogeneity of fields and the need for dedicated breast coils, magnetic resonance imaging has so far proved disappointing.

10.11 The development of breast-cancer-specific monoclonal antibodies has potential diagnostic value in all age groups either for *in vivo* scanning or to examine breast tissues or secretions.

Economic studies

10.12 Changing screening frequency, age-group screened or the screening method will all have effects on the costs and benefits of screening. An economic component should, therefore, be built into studies of these and other factors.

10.13 For better economic evaluation of the effects of breast screening further work is necessary on a definition of the quality of life appropriate to breast cancer so that realistic measures of quality-adjusted life-years can be provided.

10.14 It is assumed by some that the lower treatment costs of screen-detected breast cancer compensate for the costs of a screening programme. This assumption requires to be tested.

10.15 The comparative costs and benefits of mobile versus static units need to be defined. A research programme in the Lothians, funded by the Scottish Home and Health Department, is examining the feasibility and costs of a mobile unit.

Notification of test results

10.16 Further research is needed on the best method to inform women of the results of their screening test to ensure accuracy without causing undue anxiety.

Natural history of screen-detected cancer

10.17 It is important to determine the natural history and pathology of screen-detected breast cancer, particularly in the non-invasive phase. It is also necessary to increase our understanding of the natural history of breast cancer in younger women so that the role of screening in this age-group can be clarified.

10.18 Biological research is required into the structure and function of the normal breast, the factors that stimulate breast epithelium and their relationship to the development of cancer, for example the effect of viral and other agents.

Evaluation

10.19 To gain maximum information from a national screening programme it is necessary to have agreed and standardised protocols for the investigation and treatment of screen-detected disease, preferably within well designed studies and controlled therapeutic trials. A standardised system of recording all data, including that of pathological examination, is a prerequisite for adequate evaluation of the whole programme.

Co-ordination of research

10.20 Research will need to be co-ordinated so that duplication is avoided and merging of data facilitated. Some studies may be better conducted on a multicentre, national or UK basis. Many research needs could be met if the first centres to provide a screening service participated in co-ordinated studies.

Conclusions

10.21 Determining the optimum interval for screening must have high priority for research.

10.22 Other main areas requiring research include age, risk factors, acceptability, natural history and screening methods, with economic studies built-in where appropriate.

10.23 Adequate evaluation of a screening programme requires standardisation of recorded data.

10.24 Research should be co-ordinated. Many research needs could be met if the first centres to provide a screening service participated in co-ordinated studies.

11 Conclusions

11.1 The information already available from the principal overseas trials led us to conclude that deaths from breast cancer in women aged 50–64 years who are offered screening by mammography can be reduced by one third or more.

Basic screening methods (Chapter 4)

11.2 High-quality single medio-lateral oblique view mammography has been shown to be an effective method in reducing mortality from breast cancer and we conclude that initially this is the preferred option for the development of mass population screening.

11.3 There is no evidence that clinical examination or breast self-examination is effective when used alone. These methods may have some value when used in combination with mammography but their contribution requires further assessment.

Basic screening, selection and frequency (Chapter 5)

11.4 The effectiveness of screening has so far been demonstrated only for women aged 50 and over. In view of the poor response rates there is insufficient benefit to be gained by actively offering screening to women aged 65 or over. The priority of any screening programme should, therefore, be given to offering an initial screen to as many women as possible aged between 50–64 years. This does not exclude making screening available on demand to older women.

11.5 The use of risk factors other than age to identify women in the general population who should be screened is not practicable at present.

11.6 There is insufficient evidence on the optimum frequency for routine repeated screening and its determination must have high priority for immediate research. As a starting point for the screening programme we suggest an interval of 3 years but this must be kept under review.

Assessment, biopsy and treatment (Chapter 6)

11.7 The assessment of screen-detected abnormalities requires specialised techniques. These techniques are best carried out by a skilled multidisciplinary team, either within a hospital or in a clinic in the community. This team should consist of a clinician, a radiologist and a pathologist all trained in the diagnosis of breast disease, supported by a radiographer, a nurse and a receptionist. The availability of such teams is an essential prerequisite of a screening service for breast cancer.

11.8 Biopsies of impalpable screen-detected abnormalities should be performed, wherever possible, by a specialist breast team experienced in the surgical, radiological and pathological skills necessary for localisation techniques.

11.9 During the prevalence screen there will be an increase in the numbers to be biopsied and treated for breast cancer. While this may initially increase workload there should be a subsequent reduction to the normally expected incidence. The detection of a larger number of *in situ* cancers and small invasive cancers will favour the use of conservation techniques and this may increase certain aspects of therapeutic workload; for example, radiotherapy.

Organisation of a screening programme (Chapter 7)

11.10 While no one organisational solution for a screening programme is necessarily right for each health authority, a plan for a screening programme should include the following:

11.10.1 women in the target group should be sent a personal invitation from their general practitioner;

11.10.2 arrangements for recording positive results at the basic screen must include a fail-safe mechanism, to ensure that action is taken on all positive results;

11.10.3 every basic screening unit should have access to a specialist team for the assessment of screen-detected abnormalities;

11.10.4 a screening record system should be developed to identify, invite and recall women eligible for screening; to record attendance for screening and results; and to monitor the screening process and its effectiveness;

11.10.5 there should be adequate arrangements for quality control both within and between centres so that an acceptable standard of mammography can be maintained;

11.10.6 a designated person should be responsible for managing each local screening service. The person chosen would have managerial ability and is likely to have experience in community or preventive health care, although the radiological aspects must be the responsibility of a consultant radiologist. Setting-up a breast cancer screening service will require substantial managerial effort.

11.11 We can see considerable advantage in forming central bodies to advise Health Departments on the introduction of breast cancer screening programmes, to monitor their effectiveness and efficiency and to keep their progress under review. Such bodies might also advise their Health Departments on future policy.

Service requirements (Chapter 8)

11.12 The manpower implications for radiologists and radiographers are critical to the introduction of a screening programme. No centre should undertake screening without having a high level of expertise in mammography in order to minimise false-negative and false-positive findings.

11.13 The training of staff and the maintenance of quality is important in all relevant disciplines and for all stages in the screening procedure. The requisite expertise will need to be spread progressively from existing centres.

11.14 A basic screening unit, screening 12,000 women a year, could serve a population of some 41,500 women aged 50–64 within a total population of nearly half a million. This implies a requirement for around 120 basic units throughout the UK. This is fewer than the number of Districts and Boards in the UK (219). In view of the shortage of trained staff and the cost of equipment, it would be more cost effective, if practicable, for each basic screening unit to serve the maximum population rather than have one for each District or Board.

11.15 Specialist assessment teams should be developed in those Districts and Boards with the necessary expertise in breast cancer diagnosis, each working a sufficient number of sessions to provide for referrals from 1–3 basic screening units.

11.16 An established UK breast cancer screening programme with 120 basic screening units will require some 930 Whole Time Equivalent staff including about 40 radiologists and about 200 radiographers.

11.17 In practice, both biopsies and treatments will increasingly be concentrated on a relatively small number of surgeons and supporting assessment teams, so that any overall increase in workload will not be evenly distributed.

11.18 Training of radiologists and radiographers will have some manpower implications in the development phase of a screening programme but these should be negligible in the long-term.

11.19 Introducing a screening programme will initially require substantial capital investment in equipment and buildings. A mobile unit may, in some circumstances, be the preferred option for basic screening.

Economic appraisal (Chapter 9)

11.20 The estimates for cost per life-year or cost per QALY gained for breast cancer screening are not dissimilar to other health service activities currently undertaken. It is possible that expansion of certain other services may offer higher returns on resources spent.

11.21 We estimate that the annual revenue cost to the NHS in the UK for running a screening service, based on the Edinburgh experience and with the parameters we suggest, is about £18 million (1985–86 prices). The capital cost is likely to be at most £31 million (1985–86 prices). More frequent screening or extending the service to a much wider age range would require an increase in the number of basic units and, therefore, costs would increase *pro rata*.

Research (Chapter 10)

11.22 Determining the optimum interval for screening must have high priority for research.

11.23 Other main areas requiring research include age, risk factors, acceptability, natural history and screening methods, with economic studies built-in where appropriate.

11.24 Adequate evaluation of a screening programme requires standardisation of recorded data.

11.25 Research should be co-ordinated. Many research needs could be met if the first centres to provide a screening service participated in co-ordinated studies.

Annex A

Working Group on Breast Cancer Screening

List of members

Chairman: Professor Sir Patrick Forrest – Regius Professor of Clinical Surgery University of Edinburgh

Dr Jocelyn Chamberlain – Specialist in Community Medicine, South West Thames Regional Health Authority; and Director, DHSS Cancer Screening Evaluation Unit at the Institute of Cancer Research

Mr Arnold Elton C B E – Honorary Consultant Surgeon, Northwick Park Hospital, Middlesex

Professor Kenneth Evans (from March 1986) – Professor of Radiology, University of Wales College of Medicine

Dr Huw Gravelle (until February 1986) – Consultant Radiologist, University Hospital of Wales

Dr Dorothy Hayes – Consultant Histopathologist, Belfast City Hospital; and Honorary Lecturer, The Queen's University of Belfast

Professor Charles Joslin – Professor of Radiotherapy, University of Leeds

Ms Anne Ludbrook – Deputy Director, Health Economics Research Unit, University of Aberdeen

Dr Eric Roebuck (from March 1986) – Consultant Radiologist, University Hospital, Nottingham

Observers

Mr R Anderson – Economic Adviser's Office, DHSS

Dr D Dunstan (until December 1985) – Medical Research Council

Dr W Forbes – Scottish Home and Health Department

Mr R Greenwood (until November 1985) – Nursing Division, DHSS

Mr M Harris – Health Services Division, DHSS

Dr G Penrhyn Jones – Welsh Office

Dr F Spencer (from January 1986) – Medical Research Council

Dr H Sutton – Research Management Division, DHSS

Dr W Thornton – Department of Health and Social Services (Northern Ireland)

Miss P Wall (from December 1985) – Nursing Division, DHSS

Secretariat

Dr P Bourdillon – Medical Division, DHSS

Mr P Marshall – Health Services Division, DHSS

Ms S Novit – Health Services Division, DHSS

List of participating experts

(in alphabetical order)

Dr F Alexander, Edinburgh University

Dr T Anderson, Edinburgh University

Mrs J Andrews, Enfield District Health Authority, late Hammersmith Hospital

Ms J Ashby, Brunel University

Professor K Bagshawe, Charing Cross Hospital

Professor R Blamey, Nottingham University

Dr M Bulbrook, Imperial Cancer Research Fund

Mr M Buxton, Brunel University

Mr P Clarke, Heriot Watt University, Edinburgh

Dr J Cuzick, Imperial Cancer Research Fund

Dr J Davey, The Royal Marsden Hospital

Dr N Day, International Agency for Research on Cancer

Dr R Ellman, Institute of Cancer Research

Mr M Fitzgerald, St George's Hospital, London

Mr K Ford, King's Fund College, London

Mr N Fraser, Edinburgh University

Professor D George, University of Glasgow

Mr H Gravelle, Queen Mary College, London

Professor K Griffiths, University of Wales

Mr G Harris, Huddersfield Royal Infirmary

Dr J Hazelhurst, Marks and Spencer plc

Miss P Hibbs OBE, City and Hackney District Health Authority

Professor W Holland, St Thomas' Hospital Medical School

Professor R Jackson, University College, London

Dr A Kirkpatrick, Royal Infirmary of Edinburgh

Dr P Last, BUPA

Mr S Leinster, University of Liverpool

Dr D Mant, Oxford District Health Authority

Ms S Moss, Institute of Cancer Research

Professor D Pereira Gray, University of Exeter

Mr J Philip, Huddersfield Royal Infirmary

Dr J Price, Guildford Breast Screening, Project, Surrey

Dr M Roberts, Edinburgh Breast Screening Clinic

Dr P Skrabanek, University of Dublin

Dr C Ritchie, BUPA

Dr F Taylor, Marks and Spencer plc

Dr B Thomas, Guildford Breast Cancer Screening Project, Surrey

Professor M Vessey, University of Oxford

Professor N Wald, St Bartholomew's Hospital Mecdical School

Dr R Wrighton, Mid-Downs District Health Authority, West Sussex

Table B-1 Number of female deaths by age-group, 1985 UK

Cause of death	Age-group	0-4	5-9	10-14	15-19	20-24	25-29	30-34	35-39	40-44	45-49
Breast Cancer		-	-	-	-	7	30	113	321	506	781
All Cancers		71	65	57	90	135	201	411	936	1,312	2,180
All Causes		3,601	314	355	626	729	780	1,072	1,878	2,519	4,013

Cause of death	Age-group	50-54	55-59	60-64	65-69	70-74	75-79	80-84	85+	All ages
Breast Cancer		1,132	1,516	1,894	1,682	1,968	1,904	1,611	1,608	15,073
All Cancers		3,369	5,544	8,559	9,184	11,740	11,841	10,001	9,220	74,916
All Causes		6,568	11,697	20,313	26,040	42,465	57,156	65,289	93,679	339,094

Source: Registrar Generals; England and Wales, Scotland and Northern Ireland.

Figure B.1

Age - standardised mortality rates from breast cancer for a number of countries.
Source: World Health Statistics Annual, 1985

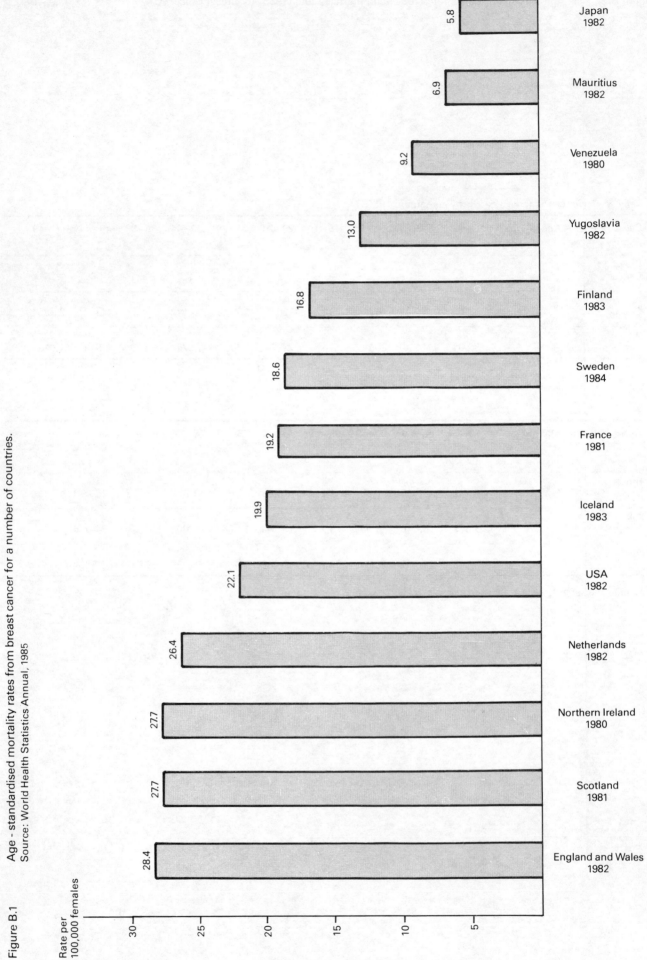

Figure B.2   Age-specific incidence rate (1982) and mortality rate (1985) for breast cancer, UK

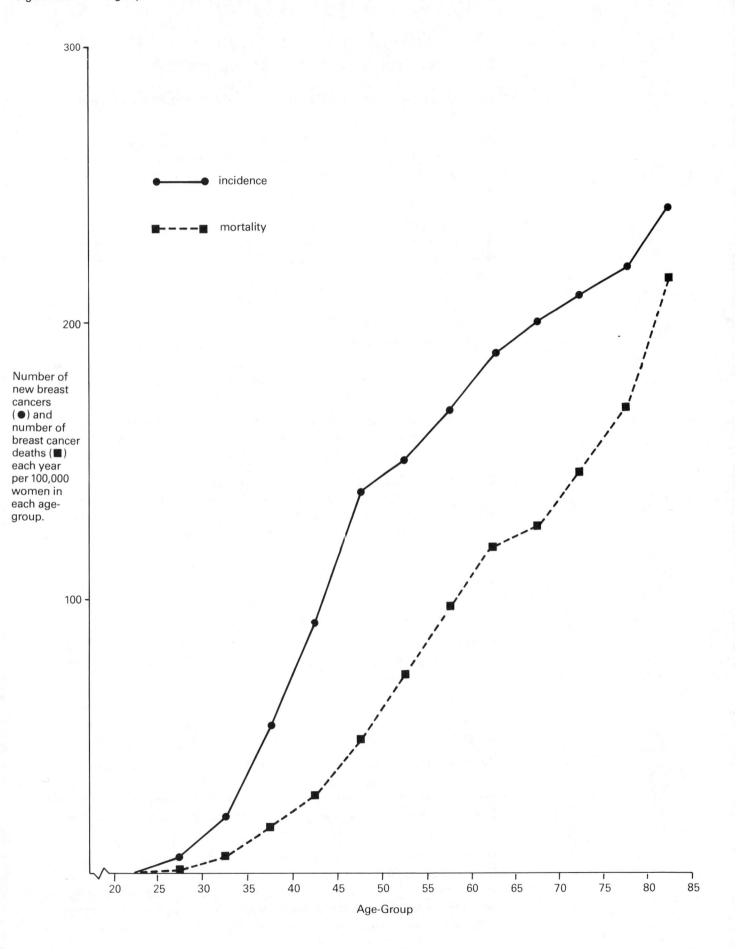

Annex C

Description of studies to evaluate the effect of screening on breast cancer mortality

C.1 **Randomised controlled trial in the Health Insurance Plan of Greater New York (HIP)**

C.1.1 **Population.** 62,000 women aged 40–64 years, with at least one year's membership of the Health Insurance Plan, were randomly allocated to a study group or a control group.

C.1.2 **Entry to programme.** December 1963–June 1966.

C.1.3 **Programme of screening.** Women in the study group were offered screening by clinical examination plus 2-view mammography at entry to the study and on three subsequent attendances at yearly intervals. The control group were not offered screening.

C.1.4 **Response.** Initial attendance was 67 per cent. Overall only 40 per cent of the study group attended all 4 screening examinations.

C.1.5 **Follow-up and definition of deaths.** Death from breast cancer is the end-point of the study. Follow-up of the entire trial population is being carried out through various sources. Deaths from breast cancer are double checked from the patients' case-notes covering the period before death.

C.1.6 **Comparability of study and control groups.** No difference was found between the groups in a number of social and demographic factors, total mortality rates (excluding breast cancer) and breast cancer incidence rates.

C.1.7 **Case detection.** A greater number of breast cancers were diagnosed at the first (prevalent) screen of the study group than arose in the first year among the control group. However, by 5 years (1 ½ years after the final offer of screening for the study group) the cumulative number of cases diagnosed since entry was similar in study and control groups and was equal at 7 years from entry. One hundred and thirty-two (43 per cent) of the 304 cases diagnosed during the first 5 years in the study group were detected by screening. There were 93 (30.6 per cent) interval cases diagnosed symptomatically after a negative screening test and 79 (36 per cent) occurred in women who had not accepted screening.

C.1.8 **Staging.** Fifty-seven per cent of cases diagnosed in the study group (71 per cent of those found by screening) had no involvement of the axillary nodes, compared with 46 per cent in the control group.

C.1.9 **Method of detection.** One third of screen-detected breast cancers were positive on mammography only and 45 per cent were positive on clinical examination only. The remaining 22 per cent were positive on both tests.

C.1.10 **Case survival.** Even allowing for one year's lead time for breast cancers diagnosed by screening, a significant improvement in survival has been maintained for study group cases over a 15-year period from diagnosis (45.7 per cent 15-year survival for the study group compared with 39 per cent for the control group).

C.1.11 **Mortality analysis.** Ten years after entry to the trial, there were 30 per cent fewer breast cancer deaths in the study group than in the control group, and after 18 years there was still a difference in favour of the study group of 23 per cent. (These comparisons apply only to deaths occurring among cases diagnosed in the first 7 years, since after this time, 3 ½ years after the final screening offer, the screening programme no longer influenced diagnosis).

C.1.12 **Effects in different age-groups.** Comparisons of the cumulative number of deaths in study and control group women in different age-groups show that among women aged over 50 years when they were first invited to be screened, a difference in favour of the study group began to appear within 3 to 5 years of entry to the programme. In younger women, however, no difference in the cumulative number of deaths was seen for more than 5 years for women aged 45 to 49 years and for more than 8 years in women aged 40 to 44 years. In women below 50 years the difference in number of deaths has never achieved statistical significance.

Sources: Selected Bibliography (31) (32) (33) (34).

C.2 Randomised Controlled Trial in Ostergötland and Kopparberg Counties, Sweden (Two Counties Study)

C.2.1 **Population.** One hundred and sixty three thousand women aged 40 years and over, resident in Ostergötland and Kopparberg counties. In Kopparberg population blocks were randomly allocated to study and control groups in a ratio of 2 to 1, in Ostergötland it was 1 to 1.

C.2.2 **Entry to programme.** 1977 to 1981.

C.2.3 **Programme of screening.** Women in the study group were offered screening by single-view mammography at entry to the study and at intervals thereafter. The rescreening interval averaged 33 months for women aged 50 years and over, and 22 months for women aged 40 years to 49 years. The control group were not offered screening although 13 per cent are known to have had at least one mammographic examination in their normal medical care.

C.2.4 **Response.** Eighty-nine per cent of women aged 40 years to 74 years accepted the initial invitation to be screened, and 83 per cent attended a second screen. In women aged 75 years and over only 50 per cent attended the initial screen. In view of the poor response in women aged over 75 years, findings are only reported for the 134,869 women under this age.

C.2.5 **Follow-up and definition of deaths.** Follow-up is through the National Bureau of Statistics. Breast cancer death certifications are verified by review of clinical and pathological records.

C.2.6 **Case detection.** After an average follow-up of 6 years from entry 1,166 breast cancers had been diagnosed in the study group and 610 in the control group. After allowing for the fact that in Kopparberg there were twice as many women in the study group as in the control group, there is a 21 per cent excess of breast cancers diagnosed in the study group.

C.2.7 **Staging.** There was a higher proportion of cancers without nodal involvement in the study group (61 per cent) compared with the controls (37 per cent). After 4 years from entry the cumulative rate of diagnosis of cancers of Stage II or more was lower in the study group than in the control group.

C.2.8 **Mortality analysis.** In the first 7 years breast cancer mortality was reduced by 31 per cent in the study group compared with the control group. The difference in cumulative mortality began to emerge 4 years after entry to the trial and has steadily widened up to 9 years. The effect was concentrated in women aged 50 and over.

Sources: Selected Bibliography (37) (38).

C.3 Population-based studies in the Netherlands: Nijmegen

C.3.1 **Population.** Thirty-thousand women aged over 35 years and resident in Nijmegen were invited for screening.

C.3.2 **Entry to programme.** January 1975 to 1982.

C.3.3 **Programme of screening.** Single-view mammography at initial attendance and repeated 3 times with a 2-year interval between each.

C.3.4 **Response.** Eighty-five per cent attended for the first screen, falling to 52 per cent by the fourth screen.

C.3.5 **Mortality analysis.** A case-control analysis was used. 'Cases' were all 46 women certified as dying of breast cancer between 1975 and 1980, whose breast cancer was diagnosed after they had been invited to attend for first screening. Each case was matched by age with 5 living residents of Nijmegen. The screening history of each case and its 5 controls was recorded up to the date of diagnosis of the case. The odds ratio of a screened woman dying of breast cancer compared to an unscreened woman was 0.48 (95 per cent confidence interval 0.23 to 1.00) indicating a possible mortality reduction of 52 per cent which was not statistically significant.

C.4 Population-based studies in the Netherlands: Utrecht

C.4.1 **Population.** Twenty thousand five hundred women aged 50 to 64 years and resident in Utrecht were invited to be screened.

C.4.2 **Entry to programme.** 1974.

C.4.3 **Programme of screening.** Clinical examination and 2-view mammography at initial attendance and on 3 subsequent occasions at intervals of 12, 18 and 24 months.

C.4.4 **Response.** Seventy-two per cent attended for initial screening.

C.4.5 **Mortality analysis.** A case-control analysis was used. 'Cases' were all 46 women who had died of breast cancer and whose breast cancer had been diagnosed after they had been invited for their first screen. Three age-matched controls who were living residents of Utrecht were selected for each case. The screening history of each case and its 3 controls was recorded up to the date of diagnosis of the case. The odds ratio of a screened woman dying of breast cancer compared with an unscreened was 0.3 (95 per cent confidence interval 0.13−0.7) indicating a statistically significant mortality reduction of 70 per cent.

C.5 Comments on Netherlands' Studies

The case-control method of analysis may be biased by self-selection of women at low risk of dying of breast cancer into the screened group. A subsidiary analysis in Nijmegen suggested no difference in the chances of *developing* breast cancer between screened and unscreened women, but it is impossible to exclude the possibility that there may have been some selection bias in their chances of *dying*. Nevertheless, the reductions in risk are large and are consistent with the results of the HIP (New York) and Two Counties (Sweden) trials so it is reasonable to conclude that part, at least, of the reduction in risk is attributable to screening. Both studies did sub-analyses by age, but with small numbers in each age-group the confidence intervals of risk estimates within age-groups were very wide and not statistically significant. In Nijmegen there was apparently no reduction in risk for women under age 50 years, and in Utrecht no reduction in risk for women aged 50−54 years.

Sources: Selected Bibliography (9) (42).

C.6 UK trials: Edinburgh randomised controlled trial

C.6.1 **Population:** Women aged 45–64 years and registered with general practitioners in Edinburgh. The general practices are randomised into a study-group and a control group.

C.6.2 **Entry to programme.** 1979 to 1981 for the initial cohort of women. Further women are added as they attain the age of 45 years.

C.6.3 **Programme of screening.** Women registered with study-group general practitioners are invited to be screened at an initial attendance and on 6 subsequent occasions at annual intervals. Screening is by clinical examination and 2-view mammography at first attendance. Thereafter, it alternates between clinical examination alone in years 2, 4 and 6 and clinical examination with single-view mammography in years 3, 5 and 7. The control group are not invited to screening, but there has been a health education campaign promoting breast awareness in the city as a whole.

C.6.4 **Response.** Sixty-three per cent of women accepted the first invitation to screening.

C.6.5 **Mortality analysis.** Information on all deaths among patients diagnosed as having breast cancer is reported and the presence of breast cancer at the time of death is verified from case-notes. The study is not yet far enough advanced to analyse the effects on mortality. The first such analysis is planned for 1987–88.

C.7 UK trials: UK Trial of Early Detection of Breast Cancer (TEDBC)

C.7.1 **Population.** Three hundred thousand women aged 45 to 64 years and registered with general practitioners serving 8 different health authorities, in Edinburgh, Guildford, Huddersfield, Nottingham, Dundee, Oxford, Southmead and Stoke.

C.7.2 **Entry to programme.** January 1979 to October 1981 for the initial cohort of women. Further women are added as they attain the age of 45 years.

C.7.3 **Programme of early detection.** The Edinburgh and Guildford populations are offered screening on 7 occasions at annual intervals. The study groups of the Edinburgh randomised controlled trial described in paragraph C.6 contributes both to that trial and to the TEDBC. Screening in Edinburgh is as described above. In Guildford screening is by clinical examination and single-view mammography at the first, third, fifth and seventh attendance, and by clinical examination alone at the second, fourth and sixth. In Huddersfield and Nottingham, all women at their entry to the trial are invited to attend a teaching session at which they are taught how and why to perform regular breast self-examination (BSE) and are encouraged to report any breast abnormalities they suspect. Self-referral diagnostic breast clinics are available for them. The remaining four populations serve as a comparison group.

C.7.4 **Response.** In Edinburgh 63 per cent and in Guildford 69 per cent of the women attended for their first screen. In Huddersfield 31 per cent and in Nottingham 50 per cent of women attended a BSE education session. The population registers used for sending out invitations were compiled from Family Practitioner Committee registers which are known to include some women who are no longer resident at the registered address. Hence the true response rates are likely to be slightly higher.

C.7.5 **Mortality analysis.** Information on deaths from breast cancer, and from all other causes, is routinely collected both by local searches in the 8 districts and by flagging the NHS Central Register record of each woman in the trial populations. The presence of breast cancer at death is verified using clinical data. The first comparison of mortality from breast cancer in the 8 populations is planned for publication in 1988.

Sources: Selected Bibliography (41) (27).

C.8 Canadian trials: Women aged 50–59 years

C.8.1 Population. Women aged 50–59 years recruited from various sources in several Canadian cities are invited to participate in a trial.

C.8.2 Entry to programme. 1980–1984.

C.8.3 Programme of screening. All of the women undergo an initial clinical examination of the breasts. Any abnormalities detected are immediately referred. The remaining women are randomly allocated to a group who are offered mammography and a group who are not. Subsequently the group offered mammography are screened by clinical examination and mammography on four successive occasions at annual intervals, and the other group are screened by clinical examination alone at the same intervals.

C.8.4 Mortality analysis. Mortality from breast cancer will ultimately be compared in the two groups.

C.9 Canadian trials: Women aged 40–49 years

C.9.1 Population. Women aged 40–49 years recruited in the same centres are invited to participate in a different trial.

C.9.2 Entry to programme. 1980–1984.

C.9.3 Programme of screening. After an initial (negative) clinical examination of the breasts, accompanied by individual education in breast self-examination, women are randomly allocated to a screening group or a control group. The screening group receive mammography and subsequently are screened by clinical examination and mammography on four successive occasions at annual intervals. The control group only receive reminders about the advisability of performing BSE.

C.9.4 Mortality analysis. Mortality from breast cancer will ultimately be compared in the two groups.

Sources: Selected Bibliography (22).

C.10 USSR trials.

The World Health Organisation is sponsoring two trials of BSE education in the USSR. In Leningrad, polyclinics are randomly divided into a study group and a control group. In Moscow, factories are similarly divided. Women registered with the study group polyclinics or working in the study group factories will be offered group education in BSE. Breast cancer incidence and mortality in study and control groups in both cities will be monitored over several years.

Source: Selected Bibliography (40).

Annex D

Radiation risk from mammography

D.1   An increased incidence of breast cancer has been observed in several groups of women exposed to high doses of radiation. These were Japanese survivors of atomic bombings at Hiroshima and Nagasaki, Canadian and American sanatoria patients who received multiple chest fluoroscopies, American women treated with radiotherapy for post-partum mastitis, Swedish women who received radiation therapy for a variety of benign breast conditions, and radium dial workers who ingested radioactive material.

D.2   This evidence also indicates that women are most at risk for the development of radiogenic breast cancer when aged less than 20 years, the risk being halved by the age of 30 and less than one tenth by the age of 40.

D.3   In the past mammography has required a relatively high dose (2–3cGy). Technical advances in recent years, especially the general use of intensifying screens, have reduced doses very substantially (typically 0.05cGy–0.15cGy), yet mammography is still too often regarded as a high dose procedure. The advent of xeromammography some years ago, with its apparent gain in image quality may have helped to perpetuate this belief, since it requires a dose about 5 or 6 times greater than mammography. However, molybdenum target tubes with molybdenum filters, used with the best film-screen combinations vacuum-packed, can now give image quality at least as good as xeromammography at much lower dose.

D.4   There is no evidence to indicate that very low doses of radiation such as those from current mammographic techniques induce breast cancer. Its existence has only been inferred from the excess breast cancer incidence seen in women exposed to higher doses. The estimated risk depends on the shape of the dose response curve in the low dose region. In a linear situation, a 10-fold reduction in exposure should lead to a 10-fold reduction in risk—the risk per cGy remains constant. In a curvilinear situation, the risk per cGy at low doses would be much less than that expected from a linear extrapolation. Most animal experiments involving a variety of radiation-induced tumours, including breast cancer, show a curvilinear relationship at low doses.

D.5   Radiogenic breast cancers in humans do not appear until a minimum of 10 years following exposure. For the years following the latent period, a risk estimate of 3.5 excess breast cancers per million women per year per cGy has been made from the Western women studied. This estimate is a linear extrapolation from high dose data due to the lack of adequate low dose data.

D.6   According to this estimate, if two million women above the age of 50 each were to receive a low dose mammogram (mean breast dose of 0.15 cGy for a single-view study) there would, after a latent period of 10 years, be one excess cancer per year in the population. This very small risk from mammography can be appreciated by comparison with the much larger magnitude of natural breast cancer incidence: 1,400 cases per million women per year at age 50 and 2,000 cases per million women per year at age 65.

D.7   Since radiation-induced and naturally-occurring breast cancers are identical pathologically, they can only be distinguished in a statistical sense. Because the risk from a dose of one cGy is so small, a 20 year follow-up of 25 million exposed and 25 million non-exposed women from age 50 would be necessary to prove or disprove risk at this level. Consequently on the evidence available, the magnitude of possible risk from low dose mammography appears negligible, especially when compared to the substantial benefits that would result from early detection.

Costs of screening methods

Unit costs of screening

E.1   From the activities at the UK trial centres, it has been possible to derive estimates of the unit costs for four basic screening methods: breast self-examination (BSE), clinical examination, mammography and mammography plus clinical examination. Estimates of the NHS cost are shown at Table E1 and the estimated costs incurred by patients are shown in Table E2.

E.2   These cost figures give a reasonable guide to the relative size of the costs involved in the different screening methods. However, the data available were not ideal. In particular, the screening programme was designed to include mammography and clinical examination every two years, with clinical examination alone in the intervening years. Therefore, costs for mammography alone have had to be estimated from the available joint costs, as have some of the clinical examination costs relating to the prevalence screen.

E.3   The time and travel costs for attending for screening in Edinburgh, shown in Table E2, have been obtained from questionnaires. These costs have been based on the assumptions that lost working time is valued at the average female wage rate, lost non-work time has been valued at 25 per cent of this rate and travel by private car has been estimated at marginal cost. Estimates produced for attending for screening in Guildford, at 1985 prices, were £1.43 per attendance for travel costs and £3.60 for time costs. In the Guildford estimates, travel by private car was estimated at full cost. Women who have any abnormality on their basic screen will, of course, attend more than once. Therefore, the average cost per woman screened would be higher.

E.4   The unit costs of the different screening methods are presented here for information but they cannot be considered in isolation. A cheaper test which detects fewer cases may not be the best choice, just as a more expensive test which detects a few extra cases may not be the best choice. Unfortunately, the data which are currently available do not allow full cost-effectiveness comparisons of the different screening methods to be made.

Marginal costs of screening

E.5   Although a complete analysis of the marginal costs and benefits of breast cancer screening is not possible from available data, the Edinburgh study has yielded some information on the marginal costs per cancer detected. Of course, the measure that is of real interest is the marginal cost per additional life year gained. Nevertheless, the figures do shed some light on the question of whether or not a combination of screening methods might be used.

E.6   Table E.3 gives estimates of the variable costs of screening by different methods; the costs included are items such as staff time and materials, while fixed costs such as buildings and equipment are excluded. (An attempt has been made to reallocate assessment costs between the different screening methods). The second column shows the estimated cancer detection rate for each method, and the final column combines the two sets of figures to give the average variable cost per cancer detected.

Table E1:   Total NHS unit cost estimates by screening method

£ 1983—84 prices

Stage in screening procedure	Cost per woman attending for:—			
	BSE	Clinical Examination	Mammography	Mammography and Clinical Examination
Basic Screen	2.57—11.44a	5.94	11.66 (single-view) 15.03 (two-view)	12.86 (single-view) 16.23 (two-view)
Assessment	b	---------------------- included in basic screen ---------------------- e			
Biopsy	b	0.57c,d	1.40c,d	2.47d
Total	2.57—11.44	6.51	13.06 (single-view) 16.43 (two-view)	15.33 (single-view) 18.70 (two-view)

Notes

a.   Per woman taught; this is sensitive to attendance rates. Average cost per session do not tend to vary.

b.   Since BSE take-up is quite low, total additional costs here may be low also.

c.   The figures for mammography and clinical examination has been calculated from data available from the prevalence screen in Edinburgh. However, the estimates for the separate modalities (clinical examination alone and mammography alone) have been based on the biopsy rates which, it was calculated, would have arisen if only one screening method had been used. There are no direct data available on the costs for single screening methods and these figures should, therefore, be viewed cautiously.

d.   Prevalence screen.

e.   It has been assumed that the assessment cost for mammography is the same as for mammography and clinical examination.

E.7   While these figures cannot be used to infer which single screening method is preferable (because they do not relate to life-years gained), they are the basis for estimating the marginal cost of adding a second screening method (as shown in Table E.4). The marginal cost of adding clinical examination to 2-view mammography is shown to be £4,643 per additional cancer detected. Similar calculations can be carried out for the addition of 2-view mammography to clinical examination and this produces a figure of £3,053 per additional cancer detected (with the assumption that the necessary equipment is already available).

Table E2:   A woman's time and travel costs per attendance

£ 1983—84 prices

	BSE	Clinical Examination	Mammography	Mammography and Clinical Examination
Travel Costs	a	0.66	0.66	0.66
Time Costs	2.37b	1.89	a	2.20

Notes

a.   Separate figures not available.

b.   Per annum; costs for one hour training and 2 hours a year carrying out monthly BSE.

Table E3: Variable cost per cancer detected

1983–84 prices

Basic Screening Method	Variable cost per 1,000 screened	Cancer detection rate (per 1,000 women screened)	Average variable cost per cancer detected
Nurse Clinical Examination*	£1,775	4.10	£ 432.9
Doctor Clinical Examination	£1,925	3.82	£ 503.9
Mammography (2-view)	£5,360	5.42	£ 988.9
Mammography and Clinical Examination	£6,660	5.70	£1,168.4

*including review by doctors when requested.

Table E4: Marginal cost calculation for adding clinical examination to mammography

1983–84 prices

Cost of mammography and clinical examination per 1 000 screened	£6,660
Cost of mammography per 1,000 screened	£5,360
Additional cost of clinical examination	£1,300
Cancers detected by mammography and clinical examination per 1,000 screened	5.70
Cancers detected by mammography per 1,000 screened	5.42
Additional cancers detected by clinical examination	0.28
Marginal cost per cancer detected by adding clinical examination	$\dfrac{£1,300}{0.28} = £4,643$

Quality assurance and quality control of mammography

F.1   Quality control within a unit and quality assurance between units are equally important. There is some overlap in the two functions. To achieve the requisite high standards there should be involvement of radiologists, radiographers and physicists with a knowledge and interest in mammographic quality.

Quality assurance

F.2   Consistent high quality results will require a quality assurance programme which may be controlled by quality assurance reference centres. Each centre would be responsible for a number of basic screening units. These centres would need to work in close liaison with each other, with interchange of material such as test films and technical results with the objective of maintaining a uniformly high standard.

F.3   Centres would be responsible for monitoring quality in established basic screening units and for testing newly marketed equipment and technical advances.

F.3.1   **Testing and evaluating newly marketed equipment and technical advances.**   Mammographic apparatus, films, screens etc need to be fully evaluated and a report prepared on suitability for use in a screening programme. Mammographic apparatus has recently been evaluated by the King's Centre for the Assessment of Radiological Equipment with the involvement of the Edinburgh, Guildford and Nottingham screening centres. Reference centres with the appropriate specialised expertise could also give an independent evaluation of technical advances (eg use of grids and rare earth filters).

F.3.2   **Monitoring quality in established units.**   Table F.1 shows the functions of a reference centre by items of equipment. Many of these items would need to be tested on a regular (daily/weekly) basis by radiographic staff at unit level under the supervision of a reference centre. Test films etc would be sent to the reference centre for comparative evaluation.

F.4   Quality control

F.4.1   **Initial testing.**   A newly installed piece of apparatus should be checked by a medical physicist to confirm the accuracy of KVp setting, beam quality, timer and automatic exposure control etc. It is important that the tube focal spot size be measured at this stage, together with the magnification function if available. The dose rate should also be checked. Similarly, film processors should be checked for developing time, temperature, replenishment rates etc.

F.4.2   **Regular testing (weekly).**   The provision of standard phantoms and film step wedges should enable radiographic staff in each unit to undertake this responsibility. From time-to-time the resulting test films would be sent to a reference centre for checking against standard results.

F.4.3   **Periodic testing.**   At intervals eg six-monthly, the mammographic apparatus needs to be re-checked by a medical physicist to ensure that no deterioration has occurred, particularly with respect to the focal spot size and the dose rate.

Table F1: Items of equipment that need testing

Mammographic Unit	Film/Screens/ Cassettes	Film Processor	Viewing Boxes/ Multiviewers	Whole System
Dose measurement.	Choice and standardisation.	Regular quality control.	Consistency of light output.	Dose calculations.
Target and filter assessment.	Screen quality checks.	Speed/contrast.	Image masking and ambient light control.	Phantom imaging.
KVp accuracy.	Cassette wear.	Basic fog levels.		Quality 'trouble shooting'.
		Solution temperatures		
Assessment of beam quality (half value layer).	Artefact identification	Chemical replenishment rates.		
Timer accuracy.				
Automatic exposure control checks.				
Light beam diaphragm alignment.				
Compression device wear.				

Film reading performance

F.5   The accuracy of basic screen film reading can be checked by sending on to the assessment stage a random sample of films classified as 'normal' intermixed with those cases genuinely referred for assessment; the interpretation of the sample films being recorded at each stage. It can also be done by interspersing films with known pathology among the films a basic screen reader has to interpret.

Radiographic performance

F.6   The accuracy of radiographic positioning, exposure etc can also be monitored by checking the random sample of films submitted for film reading performance checking.

Training of radiologists and radiographers

National organisations

G.1   At present there are two national organisations concerned with teaching mammography and general education in breast disease. These are:

G.1.1   **Symposium Mammographicum (SM).**   This is a recognised charity comprising five radiologists, one physician, two medical physicists and one radiographer formed to improve standards of mammography and to stimulate research in the subject. It has organised three national biennial symposia in London. A fourth symposium will be held in Nottingham in 1987 and will involve delegates from mainland Europe. In addition, SM has started a series of training workshops in both radiology and radiography.

G.1.2   **United Kingdom Mammographic Association (UKMA).**   This organisation was formed in 1985, as a specialist group of the Royal College of Radiologists, to bring together radiologists with an interest in mammography, to provide a forum for discussion and to stimulate teaching and research. It also provides workshop teaching particularly for radiologists involved with mammographic screening.

G.2   Training of radiologists is the responsibility of the Royal College of Radiologists, and of radiographers the College of Radiographers. Co-operation between these two bodies is being organised in the field of mammographic training. It is envisaged that the College will develop a system whereby suitable courses will be formally 'approved' by one or other body as appropriate, to ensure that the requisite standards are achieved and maintained. The courses initially will be those organised through the two national organisations. Subsequently, it is likely that, in addition, teaching centres will be set up in those undertaking mammographic screening where it is possible to accept individuals for training on secondment.

G.3   Existing programmes of teaching would need to be expanded to meet the training needs of a national population screening programme.

Training programmes

G.4   Individuals should be selected for training on the basis of an interest in screening for breast cancer and with a proven aptitude in the techniques involved. At present there are training programmes appropriate to different stages in learning and also to the intended role of the student—essentially this is the difference between mammography of symptomatic women and screening mammography. Costs are currently met by subsidies from manufacturers and delegates. The different types of training programmes are described below.

G.4.1   **Large Multidisciplinary Meetings.**   The biennial symposia organised by Symposium Mammographicum are of this type. They are attended by 300–400 delegates.

G.4.2   **Small Multidisciplinary Meetings.**   These bring together 50–60 health professionals from a number of disciplines who will be involved to some degree with mammography in order to introduce the concepts of a mammographic service for symptomatic women or for screening.

G.4.3 **Basic Workshops.** These are aimed at individuals with relatively limited experience in mammography who will be starting symptomatic mammography or who require a refresher course. They are designed to raise the level of awareness of general radiologists and radiographers in mammography and breast disease. For a national population screening programme about 5 workshops per year will be required each one catering for about 25 radiologists and about the same number for radiographers. A 2-day basic workshop costs in 1986 about £3,000.

G.4.4 **Advanced Workshops.** At present these are organised in screening centres. For a national population screening programme more centres will need to be involved. Each centre could organise about 6 workshops per year – 3 for radiologists and 3 for radiographers. A 2-day advanced workshop for 12 participants costs in 1986 about £2,000 for radiologists and £1,500 for radiographers.

G.4.5 **Individual Tuition.** For radiologists to undertake screening, two weeks secondment to a centre with experience in population screening will be required. For radiographers one weeks secondment, preferably followed by a second week after a month or two will be required. In addition to mammographic experience, individuals should be given the opportunity to attend assessment clinics, operating sessions etc. Those centres with experience in population screening will need to be provided with training facilities and will require additional manpower to allow time for teaching.

Sensitivity analysis: variations in throughput and acceptance rate

H.1 The cost figures for the basic screening unit and the implications for the NHS of introducing a national screening programme have been based on a number of assumptions. Apart from the necessary reliance upon cost data from one centre, the key elements in determining costs appear to be the throughput that can be achieved in the basic screening unit and the acceptance rate for screening.

H.2 In Chapter 8, the model for the screening programme assumed a through-put of 12,000 screens per year (including repeat films) and a population acceptance rate of 70 per cent. With one third of the population being invited for screening each year, these assumptions produced an estimate of the number of basic screening units required of around 120 (118, rounded up). Here we look at the effect of varying these assumptions.

Throughput

H.3 The throughput estimate was based on screening 30 women per session (300 per week) with the unit fully operational for an equivalent of 40 weeks (allowing for holidays, sickness, machine breakdowns etc). Taking alternative assumptions of 25 women per session (low) and 35 women per session (high) and different numbers of weeks, 38 (low) and 42 (high), produces estimates of throughput of 9,500 screens per year (low) and 14,700 (high).

Acceptance rate

H.4 The acceptance rate assumption was varied from 70 per cent by con-sidering 65 per cent (low) and 75 per cent (high). The central assumption had produced a total number of screens per year of 1,418,000; the alternative assumptions produced figures of 1,328,000 and 1,508,000.

H.5 The effect of these assumptions on the number of basic screening units required is shown in Table H.1.

H.6 The corresponding effect on the total revenue requirements of the service is shown in Table H2. It should be noted that the revenue costs per unit will vary with throughput as some of the costs are directly related to the number of women screened. The estimated costs per unit for low throughput are £125,000 per year, for the central assumption £135,000 (as given in Chapter 9) and for the high throughput, £146,000 (assuming that all costs other than overheads are avoidable).

H.7 Table H3 shows similar estimates for equipment and buildings. These vary directly in proportion to the number of basic screening units.

Table H.1: Alternative estimates of the number of basic screening units for a national programme

Total number of screens to be provided	Number of screens per unit per year		
	9,500	12,000	14,700
1,328,000	140	111	90
1,418,000	149	118	96
1,508,000	159	126	103

Table H.2: Alternative revenue estimates for a national screening programme

£m 1983–84 prices

Total number of screens to be provided	Number of screens per unit per year		
	9,500	12,000	14,700
1,328,000	17	15	13
1,418,000	19	16	14
1,508,000	20	17	15

Table H.3: Alternative equipment and buildings estimates for a national screening programme

£m 1983–84 prices

Total number of screens to be provided		Number of screens per unit per year		
		9,500	12,000	14,700
1,328,000	Equipment	16	13	10
	Buildings	17	13	11
1,418,000	Equipment	17	14	11
	Buildings	18	14	12
1,508,000	Equipment	18	14	12
	Buildings	19	15	12

Variation in screening attendances with frequency and age-group

Figure J.1   Variation in screening attendances with frequency and age-group.

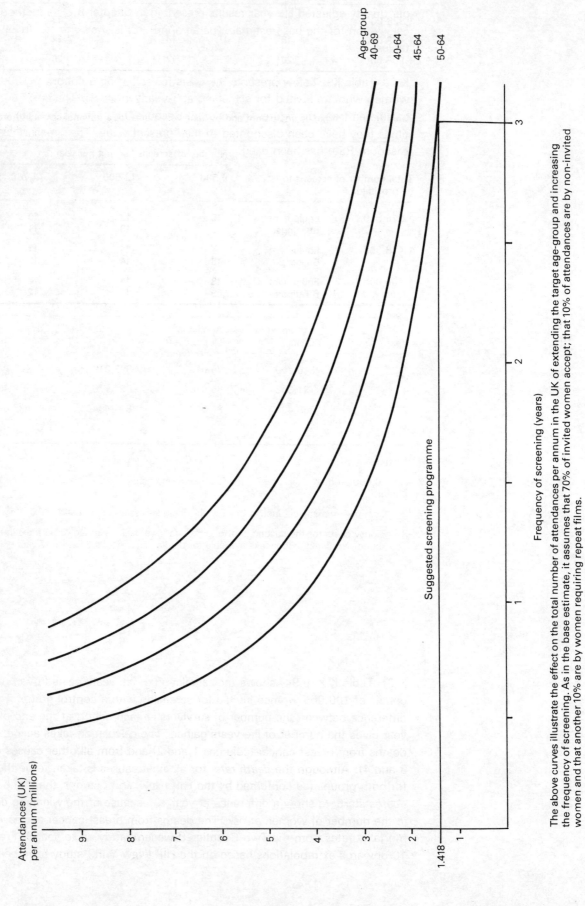

Attendances (UK)
per annum (millions)

Age-group
40-69
40-64
45-64
50-64

Suggested screening programme

Frequency of screening (years)

The above curves illustrate the effect on the total number of attendances per annum in the UK of extending the target age-group and increasing the frequency of screening. As in the base estimate, it assumes that 70% of invited women accept; that 10% of attendances are by non-invited women and that another 10% are by women requiring repeat films.

Annex K

Cost per life-year calculations

K.1 This annex presents the details that underlie the cost per life-year and cost per quality-adjusted life-year results presented in Chapter 9. The method of calculation for the base estimate (paragraph 9.26) is shown in the following tables.

K.2 Table K.1 below presents the costs for screening a cohort of 100,000 women who are invited for screening at 3-yearly intervals. The costs are calculated from the figures in Annex E. Because the costs occur at different times they have been discounted to their present value. The Treasury Test Discount Rate has been used.

Table K.1 Cost of the screening programme for an invited population of 100,000 women.

£ 1983–84 prices

Year	Screening Costs	Additional biopsy costs	Total	Discounted at 5% per annum
1	816,200	86,018	902,218	902,218
4	791,958	86,018	877,976	758,429
7	768,436	86,018	854,454	637,607
				2,298,254

Notes

1. 70,000 women attend first screening round; attendance reduces at a rate of 1 per cent per annum.

2. Cost per woman screened is £11.66; this includes assessment costs.

3. Biopsy costs for the second and third rounds have been assumed to be the same as for the first round. No direct evidence is available for biopsy rates after a 3-year interval.

K.3 Table K.2 (p.94) shows the calculation of life-years gained by comparing a cohort of 100,000 women invited for screening with a control group. The difference between the number of survivors in each cohort at the end of each year gives the number of life-years gained. The calculation takes account of deaths from breast cancer (columns 1 and 2) and from all other causes (columns 3 and 4). Although the *death rate* for all other causes is taken to be the same for both groups (as confirmed by the HIP (New York) study), the number of *deaths* starts to show a difference at year 10 because of the widening difference in the number of women at risk. The deaths from breast cancer are based on mortality rates from the Two Counties (Sweden) study up to year 9. From year 10 onwards extrapolations based on the HIP (New York) study have been used.

Table K.2 Life-years gained for a cohort of 100,000 women invited for screening compared with a control group.

Year	Deaths from breast cancer		Deaths from all other causes		Population surviving		Life-years gained (difference of columns 5 and 6) (7)
	Invited for screening (1)	Control (2)	Invited for screening (3)	Control (4)	Invited for screening (5)	Control (6)	
					100,000	100,000	
1	2.82	5.63	573	573	99,424	99,421	3
2	11.23	21.75	570	570	98,843	98,830	13
3	26.56	23.72	566	566	98,250	98,240	10
4	22.23	19.40	563	563	97,665	97,658	7
5	27.65	54.07	560	560	97,078	97,043	35
6	34.43	51.67	556	556	96,487	96,436	51
7	50.14	58.96	553	553	95,884	95,824	60
8	29.87	61.37	549	549	95,305	95,213	92
9	33.76	66.45	546	546	94,725	94,601	124
10	45.6	61.4	543	542	94,136	93,998	138
11	57.3	56.5	539	539	93,540	93,403	137
12	56.9	56.1	536	535	92,947	92,812	135
13	56.6	55.8	533	532	92,357	92,224	133
14	56.2	55.4	529	528	91,772	91,641	131
15	33.9	34.7	526	525	91,212	91,081	131

K.4 The life-years gained by screening occur at different points in time, as do the costs. The same discounting procedure is therefore applied to these benefits. The calculation is shown in Table K.3 below.

K.5 The cost per life-year gained is given by dividing the discounted cost of the screening programme, £2,298,254 (from Table K.1), by the discounted life-years gained, 755.02 (from Table K.3). This gives £3,044 per life-year gained, as given in paragraph 9.26.

Table K.3 Discounting the life-years gained.

Year	Life-years gained	Discounted at 5% per annum	Cumulative discounted life-years gained
1	3	3	3
2	13	12.38	15.38
3	10	9.07	24.45
4	7	6.05	30.50
5	35	28.79	59.29
6	51	39.96	99.25
7	60	44.77	144.02
8	92	65.38	209.40
9	124	83.93	293.33
10	138	88.96	382.29
11	137	84.11	466.40
12	135	78.93	545.33
13	133	74.06	619.39
14	131	69.47	688.86
15	131	66.16	755.02

Selected Bibilography

1. ADAM, S (1982). The effect of a breast self-examination campaign in Daventry. MD Thesis, University of Edinburgh.

2. ARON, JL AND PROROK, PC (1986). An analysis of the mortality effect in a breast cancer screening study. Internatinal Journal of Epidemiology 15, 1, 36-43.

3. BEAHRS, OH, SHAPIRO, S, SMART, C AND MCDIVITT, MD (1979). Report of the working group to review the National Cancer Institute – American Cancer Society breast cancer detection demonstration projects. Journal of the National Cancer Institute 62, 647-709.

4. BULBROOK, RD, MOORE, JW, CLARK, GMG, WANG, DY, MILLIS, RR AND HAYWARD, JL (1986). Relation between risk of breast cancer and biological availability of estradiol in the blood. Annals of the New York Academy of Science 464, 378-388.

5. CALNAN, MW, CHAMBERLAIN, J AND MOSS, S (1983). Compliance with a class teaching breast self-examination. Journal of Epidemiology and Community Health 37, 264-270.

6. CHAMBERLAIN, J (1985). Secondary prevention: screening for breast cancer. Effective Health Care 2, 179-187.

7. CHAMBERLAIN, J, CLIFFORD, RE, NATHAN, BE, PRICE, JL AND BURN, I (1984). Repeated screening for breast cancer. Journal of Epidemiology and Community Health 38, 54-57.

8. CLARKE, PR AND FRASER, N (1986). An economic analysis of breast cancer screening. Health Economists Study Group Meeting, University of Bath.

9. COLETTE, HJA, DAY, NE, ROMBACH, JJ AND DE WAARD, F (1984). Evaluation of screening for breast cancer in a non-randomised study (the DOM project) by means of a case control study. Lancet 1, 1224-26.

10. DUFFY, SW, ROBERTS, MM AND ELTON, RA (1983). Risk factors for breast cancer: relevance to screening. Journal of Epidemiology and Community Health 37, 127-131.

11. DUPONT, WD AND PAGE, DL (1985). Risk factors for breast cancer in women with proliferative breast disease. The New England Journal of Medicine 312, 146-151.

12. FRANK, JW, AND MAI, V (1985). Breast self-examination in young women: more harm than good? Lancet 2, 654-657.

13. GOHAGAN, JK, DARBY, WP, SPITZNAGEL, EL, MONSEES, BS AND TOME, AE (1986). Radiogenic breast cancer effects of mammographic screening. Journal of the National Cancer Institute 77, 71–76.

14. GRAVELLE, IH, BULSTRODE, JC, BULBROOK, RD AND HAYWARD, JL (1986). A prospective study of mammographic parenchymal patterns and risk of breast cancer. British Journal of Radiology 59, 701, 487–491.

15. GRAVELLE, HSE, SIMPSON, PR AND CHAMBERLAIN, J (1982). Breast cancer screening and health service costs. Journal of Health Economics 1, 185–207.

16. HAKANSSON, S AND JONSSON, E (1984). Screening for cancer – underlaget däligt för kalkyl om kostnader och nytta. Läkartidningen 81, 4734–4742.

17. HUTCHINSON, J AND TUCKER, AK (1984). Breast screening results from a healthy working population. Clinical Oncology 10, 123–128.

18. JONSSON, E AND HAKANSSON, S (1986). Ekonomisk a konsekvenser av mammografisk hälsokontroll – en översikt. Läkartidningen 83, 22, 2050–2053.

19. KALACHE, A AND VESSEY, M (1982). Risks factors for breast cancer. Clinics in Oncology 1, 661–678.

20. KOPANS, DB, MEYER, JE AND SADOWSKY, N (1984). Breast imaging. The New England Journal of Medicine 310, 960–967.

21. LAST, PA, RITCHIE, CD AND WILLIS, L (1985). The Well Woman Clinic. Journal of Obstetrics and Gynaecology 5, Supplement 2, S78–S82.

22. MILLER, AB, HOWE, GR AND WALL, C (1981). The national study of breast cancer screening. Protocol for a Canadian randomised controlled trial of screening for breast cancer in women. Clinical Investigative Medicine 4, 227–258.

23. MOORE, JW, CLARK, GMG, BULBROOK, RD, HAYWARD, JL, MURAI, JT, HAMMOND, GL AND SIITERI, PK (1982). Serum concentrations of total and non-protein-bound oestradiol in patients with breast cancer and in normal controls. International Journal of Cancer 29, 17–21.

24. MOSKOWITZ, M AND GARSIDE, P (1982). Evidence of breast cancer mortality reduction: Aggresive screening in women under age 50. American Journal of Radiology 138, 911–916.

25. NICHOLLS, S AND WATERS, W E (1982). The effect on doctor's workload of a campaign to encourage the early reporting of breast symptoms. Journal of Epidemiology and Community Health 36, 228–230.

26. REPORT OF THE COUNCIL ON SCIENTIFIC AFFAIRS. (1984). Early detection of breast cancer. Journal of the American Medical Association 252, 3008–3011.

27. ROBERTS, MM, ALEXANDER, FE, ANDERSON, TJ, FORREST, APM, HEPBURN, W, HUGGINS, A, KIRKPATRICK, AE, LAMB, J, LUTZ, W AND MUIR, BB (1984). The Edinburgh randomised trial of screening for breast cancer: description of method. British Journal of Cancer 50, 1–6.

28. ROBERTS, MM, JONES, V, ELTON, RA, FORTT, RW, WILLIAMS, S AND GRAVELLE, IH (1984). Risk of breast cancer in women with history of benign disease of the breast. British Medical Journal 288, 275–278.

29. ROEBUCK, EJ (1986). Mammography and screening for breast cancer. British Medical Journal 292, 223–226.

30. ROMBACH, JJ, COLLETTE, BJA, DE WAARD, F AND SLOTBOOM, BJ, (1986). Analysis of the diagnostic performance in breast cancer screening by relative operating characteristics. Cancer 58, 169–177.

31. SHAPIRO, S, STRAX, P AND VENET, L (1971). Periodic breast cancer screening in reducing mortality from breast cancer. Journal of the American Medical Association 215, 1777–1785.

32. SHAPIRO, S (1977). Evidence on screening for breast cancer from a randomized trial. Cancer 39, 2772–2782.

33. SHAPIRO, S, VENET, W, STRAX, P, VENET, L AND ROESER, R (1982). Ten- to fourteen-year effect of breast cancer screening on mortality. Journal of the National Cancer Institute 69, 349–355.

34. SHAPIRO, S (1986). Paper presented to UICC Workshop on screening for breast cancer, Helsinki.

35. TABAR, L AND DEAN, PB (1982). Mammographic parenchymal patterns. Journal of the American Medical Association 247, 185–189.

36. TABAR, L AND GAD, A (1981). Screening for breast cancer – the Swedish trial. American Journal of Radiology 138, 219–222.

37. TABAR, L, GAD, A, HOLMBERG, LH, LJUNGQUIST, U, EKLUND, G, PETTERSSON, F, FAGERBERG, CJG, BALDETORP, L, GRONTOFT, O, LUNDSTROM, B, MANSON, JC AND DAY, NE (1985). Reduction in mortality from breast cancer after mass screening with mammography. Randomised trial from the Breast Cancer Screening Working Group of the Swedish National Board of Health and Welfare. Lancet 1, 829–832.

38. TABAR, L (1986). Paper presented to UICC Workshops on screening for breast cancer, Helsinki.

39. TORRANCE, GW (1986). Measurement of health state utilities for economic appraisal. Journal of Health Economics 5, 1–30.

40. TSECHKOVSKI, M, SEMIGLASOV, V, SAGAIDASK, V, MOISEYENKO, V AND MIKHAILOV, E (1986). Role of breast self-examination in reduction of mortality from breast cancer. Protocol of the study, WHO.

41. UK TRIAL OF EARLY DETECTION OF BREAST CANCER GROUP. (1981). Trial of early detection of breast cancer: description of method. British Journal of Cancer 44, 618–627.

42. VERBEEK, ALM, HENDRICKS, JHCL, HOLLAND, R, MRAVUNAC, M, STURMANS, F AND DAY, NE (1984). Reduction of breast cancer mortality through mass screening with modern mammography. First results of the Nijmegen Project, 1975–1981. Lancet 1, 1222–1224.

43. WANG, D Y AND FENTIMAN, I S (1985). Epidemiology and endocrinology of benign breast disease. British Cancer Research and Treatment 6, 5–36.

44. WERTHEIMER, M D, COSTANZA, M E, DODSON, T F, D'ORSI, C, PASTIDES, H AND ZAPKA, J G (1986). Increasing the effort toward breast cancer detection. Journal of the American Medical Association 255, 1311–1315.

45. WHITEHEAD, J, CARLILE, T, KOPECKY, K J, THOMPSON, D J, GILBERT, JR, FI, PRESENT, A J, THREATT, B A, KROOK, P AND HADAWAY, E (1986). The relationship between Wolfe's classification of mammograms, accepted breast cancer risk factors, and the incidence of breast cancer. American Journal of Epidemiology 122, 994–1006.

46. WILLIAMS, A (1985). Economics of coronary artery bypass grafting. British Medical Journal 291, 326–329.

47. WILSON, J M G AND JUNGNER, G (1968). Principles and practice of screening for disease. World Health Organisation. WHO Public Health Paper, 34.

48. ZUUR, C AND BROERSE, J J (1985). Risk – and cost-benefit analysis of breast screening programs derived from absorbed dose measurements in the Netherlands, XIV ICMBE and VII ICMP, Espoo, Finland 520–521.

Glossary

Acceptance Rate

The proportion of those invited for screening who accept.

Benign Breast Disease

Breast cells which have a minor abnormality but which are not malignant and do not have the potential for spread.

Biopsy

Removal of a small piece of tissue for laboratory examination by a pathologist to determine whether it is malignant.

Breast Self-Examination (BSE)

The regular examination (eg monthly) of the breasts by the woman herself.

Chemotherapy

Use of one or more anti-cancer drugs to destroy cancer cells which have spread from the original site. Also used as back-up to primary treatment (usually, surgery) of breast cancer, with the intention of destroying undetected foci of cells which may have already spread.

Clinical Examination

Clinical examination of the breast is the physical examination of the breast by trained medical or nursing personnel.

Cost-Benefit Analysis (CBA)

An analysis of all the costs and benefits of any proposal, ideally expressed in commensurate (ie money) terms. If the costs exceed the benefit then the proposal is not justified on economic grounds.

Cost-Effectiveness Analysis (CEA)

An analysis of the costs of achieving a given end. The most cost-effective method is the one that produces the required outcome at least cost (or which maximises the beneficial outcome from a fixed budget).

Cost-Utility Analysis (CUA)

A form of *CBA*, developed in the health field, in which changes in health status are considered explicity and not converted to monetary values. All other costs and benefits are treated as in *CBA*. Results are usually expressed in terms of cost per life-year gained or cost per *quality-adjusted-life-year gained (QALY)*.

Cyst

A sac with a distinct wall containing fluid or semisolid matter.

Cytology

Microscopic examination of individual or groups of cells.

Excision Biopsy

Surgical removal of a portion of tissue for examination by a pathologist. The procedure may be done under general or local anaesthetic. The laboratory processing and examination of the tissue takes 1 to 2 days.

Fine Needle Aspiration

A technique used to differentiate cystic from solid lesions in the breast. A needle is inserted in the lesion and the material drawn out using a syringe. If the material is solid it can be stained and the cells examined in a laboratory to determine whether the cells are benign or malignant. This is known as *Fine Needle Aspiration Cytology*.

Frozen Section Biopsy

Surgical removal of a portion of tissue for immediate examination by a pathologist. The laboratory freezes the specimen to enable it to be sectioned and examined microscopically within a few minutes of its removal. The usual reason for doing this procedure is to enable diagnosis and further surgical treatment to be done under the same anaesthetic.

Histological Examination

The microscopic study of tissues removed from the body.

Hormone Therapy

Treatment by hormones. Used as back-up to primary treatment (usually, surgery) of breast cancer.

Impalpable Tumours

Tumours that are not detectable by touch.

Incidence

The number of newly diagnosed cases of disease in a defined population within a defined time period. It is usual to present incidence as rates per 100,000 eg a breast cancer incidence rate of 200 per 100,000 females per year, means that there are 200 new cases of breast cancer each year for every 100,000 women in the population.

Incident Screen

Any screen a person has after the first screen. It detects incident disease ie that which has arisen since the previous screen.

Interval Cancer

A cancer that is diagnosed because of symptoms within a stated interval after a negative screening test.

Lead-Time

The time between the date of detection of a cancer by screening and the date when it would have been diagnosed if the patient had not been screened. Survival is measured from the time of diagnosis, but screening advances the date at which diagnosis is made, thus automatically lengthening the survival time even if it makes no difference to the date of death. This is known as *lead-time bias*.

Length-Bias	The tendency for screening to detect a disproportionate number of cancers which spend a long time in the preclinical detectable phase. By implication a long duration in this phase suggests that these cancers are relatively slow growing and have a good prognosis.
Lesion	Any pathological change in a bodily tissue.
Lymph Node	Small accumulation of normal glandular tissue where lymph is purified and lymphocytes are formed. In breast cancer the condition of local lymph nodes indicates whether the disease has spread beyond the breast.
Malignant Cells	Cancer cells which have the potential to spread.
Mammography	X-ray examination of the breast.
Menarche	Age at which the menstrual periods first start.
Menopause	Ending of menstruation, signifying the end of a woman's reproductive life. Normally takes place between the ages of 45 and 55.
Metastases	Secondary cancer deposits which have detached themselves from the primary tumour and in the case of breast cancer have spread to local *lymph nodes* and/or distant sites such as the bones, liver and brain.
Mortality	The number of people in a defined population who die within a defined time period. As for *incidence* it is usual to present mortality as rates per 100,000.
Pathologist	Specialist in laboratory medicine concerned with identifying the changes in body tissues and organs which cause or are caused by disease.
Prevalence	The total number of cases of disease present in a defined population at any one time.
Prevalence screen	The first screen a person has, which picks up all the prevalent disease which may have accumulated up to that time.
Prognosis	A forecast of the probable course and outcome of a disease.
Quality-adusted-life-year (QALY)	This is an outcome measure which combines changes in life expectancy as the result of any intervention (life-years gained) with the expected morbidity or quality of life associated with those life-years. It is recognised that comparing the outcomes of different health service interventions only in terms of life-years gained is inappropriate because it is not comparing like with like. Techniques for assessing the relative weight to be given to different types of morbidity are being developed and quality adjustment values should be seen as indicative at this stage.

Radiographer　　Professionally trained person who takes radiographs and is involved with other imaging techniques.

Radiologist　　Specialist concerned with the diagnosis of disease by means of imaging techniques.

Radiotherapy　　Treatment of cancer by X-rays and other forms of radiation to destroy the malignant cells.

Rosser Scaling　　A technique developed by Rosser and Kind for estimating quality-of-life adjustments. *(See QALY)*. Their approach classifies health states on two dimensions; physical disability and distress. Relative weights to attach to each health state were obtained after detailed interviewing of a sample of 70 subjects.

Selection Bias　　The tendency for people who accept screening to be atypical of the population from which they come.

Sensitivity　　The ability of a test to detect a disease; a test with a sensitivity of 90% will give a positive result in 9 out of 10 cases of disease present in the screened people.

Specificity　　The ability of a test to exclude people who do not have disease; a test with a specificity of 90% will give a negative result in 900 out of 1,000 non-diseased people who are screened.

Survival Rate　　The proportion of patients with a disease who are alive at a given time after diagnosis (or treatment).

Tumour　　Swelling or mass of abnormal tissue. Often used as a synonym for cancer although strictly speaking not all tumours are malignant.

Ultrasonography　　Production of a visual image of deep structures of the body by recording the echoes of sound waves directed into the tissues.

Printed in the United Kingdom for Her Majesty's Stationery Office.
Dd.0291378, 3/89, C15, 3385/4, 5673, 54383.